Food
Freedom
And Truth

How to Stop Following Your Thoughts and
Feelings to the Refrigerator

Laura Katleman

Cave of the Heart Publishing

Cave of the Heart Publishing

ISBN: 978-1477544785

Copyright © 2012 by Laura Katleman

Change the Lenses of your Glasses
I Robot

THE TRUTH ABOUT ENDING EMOTIONAL EATING

Changing Perception is the Key to Transformation
Relationship with Thoughts
Where's the Benefit?
Your Achilles Heels
Stressful Thoughts and Emotional Eating
Living as a Human Being Meditation
The Fun Factor
Repression and Living and Speaking from Your Heart
Junk Food for the Mind
Healing Emotional Eating
What If We Have It All Wrong?
End of Life Meditation

THE TRUTH ABOUT HAPPINESS

What World Do You Want to Live in?
What Are You Loving?
Being Present with Food
The Ego's Relationship to Eating
Playing
Support
The Pleaser Disease
Asking for Support
The Short Cut to True Happiness
Four Ways To Weaken Conditioning
A Gratitude Attitude

For Richard Gage and all the other heroes throughout history who took a courageous stand for freedom and truth.

ACKNOWLEDGMENTS

If these pages contain any wisdom, it comes from the "deep wells" I call my teachers, specifically Gina Lake, Stuart Schwartz, Pamela Wilson, Mooji, Michael Regan, Neelam, Adyashanti, Byron Katie, Eckhart Tolle, Ramana Maharshi, Robert Adams, Krishnamurti, Yogananda, and Nisargadatta. I thank them. I would also like to thank those I have not called teacher but who, nevertheless, have had a profound impact on loosening my ties of identification with the ego: my ex husbands, my daughter, our dog, my parents and sisters, my friends, and the greatest teacher of all—life. I bow to all of you in deep reverence and gratitude. I hope that in some small measure this book will also serve the freedom of those who read it and put it into practice.

Food Freedom And Truth

INTRODUCTION

Food, Freedom and Truth explores the human condition through the lens of a challenging relationship with food and focuses on our ability to wake up from our programming and live life from the natural state. Our relationship with food and, ultimately, our entire experience of life boil down to one thing: how we respond to our thoughts. When we see this truth, we can choose to ignore our thoughts rather than follow them, move with life instead of resist it and stop creating the negative feelings that keep us running to the refrigerator.

In these pages, you will learn that (1) feelings are not random occurrences, erupting willy-nilly without your consent—you create them; (2) by choosing to stop creating negative feelings, you don't have to live at their effect; and (3) you select your experience of life depending on what you believe and where you put your attention.

A misalignment with food is a spiritual issue. We eat too much and eat the wrong foods because we are unhappy and unwittingly creating negative feelings. This pattern of eating to get happy becomes a self-reinforcing cycle. If we're unhappy, we eat too much and gain weight, causing us to feel worse about ourselves. The unhappier we become, the more we are likely to try to get relief through food. In other words, when eating is our habitual way of coping with unhappy feelings, we turn to food for relief and, in doing so, exacerbate the problem.

Telling Yourself the Truth

Emotional eating is problematic not just because it can negatively impact your health, but because it means that you're romanticizing food—looking for it to provide comfort, diversion or entertainment. This belies a misunderstanding about the true function of food as fuel. In addition, emotional eating points to an innocent misunderstanding of how to *live*. Most of us have never learned how to be happy or, more accurately , how to avoid being unhappy. As crazy as it sounds, human beings are programmed to be unhappy because we are conditioned to listen to and believe our negative thoughts. And whenever we buy into the whingeing of a negative mind, we unconsciously generate unhappy feelings.

In the upcoming pages, you will learn to turn this pattern around by uncovering and stymieing the unconscious habit of generating negative feelings. When you stop buying into negative thoughts and stop creating negative feelings, you live life at a higher vibration. You may live in the same place with the same family and friends, but you truly live in a different world—a heaven on earth.

Unfortunately, for most people, life on earth is anything but heavenly. Unaware that they have a choice in the matter, most people live at the effect of their feelings. They continually create negative feelings, and stay locked up in egoic consciousness, a place of contraction and resistance to life. Living from this place reinforces the programmed misunderstanding that we are separate human beings with stressful thoughts and feelings that deserve attention and validation. Holding the perspective that we are all separate people competing for limited resources is how we create fear, mistrust the goodness of life and see other people as the enemy. It's how we keep ourselves from the truth of the one consciousness that connects all of our hearts, and how we innocently cause our own unhappiness. It's how we create war inside ourselves and with others.

When we realize that we can choose to create negative feelings or not, we stand our world on end, dramatically impacting our happiness. How wonderful to realize that as creators of positive feelings, rather than victims of random ones that arrive unbidden, we have the power to radically shift and elevate our own consciousness.

Some people would assert that there are two selves: a higher, or virtuous, one and a lower, or egoic, one. The higher one upholds the high opinion we have of ourselves while the lower one justifies the poor opinion we have of ourselves. But the truth is that there has only ever been one of us, the single being that I call *essence,* which peers out through all of our eyes and is the epitome of love, kindness, humility, gratitude and compassion.

So what of the ego, then? Is it real or did we make it up? We give a name to the ego as if it's really a thing, but in fact it has never actually existed. It's just what we call an idea that serves as a container for all of our judgmental, resistant and fearful notions about other people, life and ourselves. Yet, for our purpose—waking up from our misguided, painful relationship with food, weight and our bodies—we will pretend that the ego does exist.

We might describe the ego as *the false self,* a bundle of erroneous thoughts that we have come to believe over the years. These beliefs, often referred to as *conditioning,* can profoundly impact our choices and quality of life. If we can uncover and question them, we can see them as the lies they have always been, and unlock their stranglehold on our happiness.

The sections in *Food, Freedom and Truth* are organized into seven main parts: Telling Yourself the Truth; The Truth About Desire; The Truth About Beliefs; The Truth About Emotions; The Truth About Bodies; The Truth About Ending Emotional Eating; and The Truth About Happiness. Each section deals with a different facet of the misunderstanding that holds our food, weight and body-image issues in place. Illuminating these areas helps us to see through the broken places in ourselves and heal the negative beliefs that keep us bound.

Read this book slowly, perhaps just one section at a time. As you move through the book, you will walk the path traversed by seekers for time immemorial, free yourself from your food prison, wake up out of identification with your ego and melt back into essence, the true spiritual self.

TELLING YOURSELF THE TRUTH

We empower thoughts and give them life until they appear to have a life of their own. When we stop giving the thoughts energy, they settle. While we give thoughts our life energy, they grow into worlds and we believe certain thoughts are who we are and certain thoughts are not who we are. Then we have likes and dislikes, or things we desire and things we resist. When we can allow thoughts to just be and allow emotions to just be, then they settle and a feeling arises that was being covered by the thoughts and emotions. This is not something we like or dislike, it is the feeling of being, which is natural and effortless.

Ramana Maharshi

The Truth About Emotional Eating

If you are reading these words because food has become the moon and the stars and the setting sun for you, you are in the right place. The wonderful news about emotional eating is that it is a habit. And like any other habit, you formed it through repetition over time and you can undo it through repeated effort over time. Unlike alcoholism, emotional eating is not a disease. It can feel like a vexing affliction, but you don't have to accept the label of emotional eater for life. You don't need to attend daily or weekly meetings, call a sponsor or admit to yourself or God that you are powerless around food.

Don't get me wrong. Many people have managed their emotional eating using these tools. But in my experience, it is possible to *heal* emotional eating for good, not just manage it, and get on about the business of living without worrying that the next emotion you feel will send you face-first into a pint of ice cream.

In fact, not only is healing possible, it's the likely outcome of using awareness exercises, guided meditation and *inquiry*, a tool for questioning the stressful beliefs that cause suffering, all of which you will learn about in the upcoming pages. Healing emotional eating is a maturation process, which means that once you begin, your healing is inevitable and irreversible.

This may seem hard to believe, but I promise you, most people who knew me as a raging food addict would have told you that curing my emotional eating in this lifetime was about as likely as a snowstorm in Tahiti. As an emotional eater, I used to reach for food in response to changes in my emotional state, like boredom, stress or sadness. Anything that moved me off my equilibrium or stasis generally caused me to run to the refrigerator. Even positive emotions like excitement and happiness could trigger emotional eating.

I first formed my emotional connection with food in childhood, after fighting with my sister, which was a daily occurrence. Whenever I felt dejected and unsupported by my parents, I'd head to the freezer for a huge slab of chocolate ice cream and march to a room at the back of the house, where I'd switch on the television. Distracted by the story line of a sitcom, within a matter of minutes, I'd no longer feel angry. On some level, I must have attributed my inner calm to the ice cream, rather than to the fact that I was no longer fuming and thinking about how unfair my sister and parents were. And from childhood until my late forties, I turned to food hoping it could remove my emotional suffering.

We eat emotionally because we formed a belief during childhood that eating has the power to distract us from or numb our feelings. Yet the actual experience of emotional eating doesn't bear this out. Here is what actually happens: All of a sudden, for no apparent reason, you feel an uncontrollable urge to eat something. At this point, you may or may not be aware that you are in the throes of an emotion. You seek out starchy, fatty or sweet food and start shoveling in bites as fast as you can.

Your premise may be that you are eating to avoid feeling an emotion, and that may happen for a few moments. But emotional eating is actually eating unconsciously *while* you are feeling and thinking at the same time. The emotion is still present after your emotional eating episode, but by then, you have added shame, regret, bloating, disappointment and potential weight gain to your original emotional discomfort. So not only does emotional eating fail to keep you from feeling an emotion, the act itself packs an emotional punch and actually adds to your emotional burden.

Having spent almost half a century trying to overcome my eating issues, I finally understand why healing a misalignment with food can be such a challenge. Unlike other addictive substances, we need food to survive. We can't just swear off it and say, "I've had it with this troublesome food stuff." Our choices are to abstain and die, live with our dysfunctional relationship and continue to suffer, or declare that we're fed up and resolve to do whatever it takes to heal our relationship with food once and for all.

Eating issues are complex and multifaceted, and the challenges they present vary from person to person. For example, a while ago one of my clients told me that she had become aware that she wasn't speaking up for herself. After taking an assertiveness-training class, her food issues went away. Another client told me she was force-fed as a child when she refused to eat something. She got so angry at her mother that she told her she hated her. As an adult, her guilt over talking to her mother that way manifested as binge eating. Every time she was in a situation she didn't like but felt powerless to change, she punished herself for the anger she felt about it by bingeing. Another client told me that he noticed he was getting home in the afternoon and making a beeline to the refrigerator. One day, he asked himself if he was experiencing physical hunger. He realized that he wasn't, and asked himself, "What's going on here?" It occurred to him that he was tired, and instead of eating, he took a nap. Afternoon naps became his new habit. From that change alone, he lost 10 pounds.

Food Freedom And Truth

In general, a misalignment with food is a spiritual and lifestyle misalignment. If you aren't happy and are constantly trying to get happy through food, healing requires that you ask yourself some tough questions.

Exercise: Lifestyle Inquiry

Ask yourself the following questions and record your answers in a journal. As you live your life over the next few days, keep these questions in mind, and continue to refine your answers. Then, make any changes that seem warranted.

❖ How am I living? Am I aligned with my life purpose?

❖ Am I expressing what's true for me, both verbally and in my actions?

❖ Am I taking care of myself emotionally and physically? Am I getting enough rest and taking time to feed my soul?

❖ Am I questioning the stressful thoughts and beliefs that cause me to suffer? Or am I continuing to weave painful stories?

Telling Yourself the Truth

If you are truly ready to hop off the treadmill of eating-related misery, you need to ask yourself these questions, tell yourself the truth and make changes in your life based on the answers. If you're not speaking up or standing up for yourself, change that, even if it means taking an assertiveness-training class to help you learn how. If your lifestyle doesn't suit you, begin to make decisions that support your happiness. Even making a small change will help. Use inquiry to question the stressful beliefs that have been running your life. Realize that they never tell the whole truth, and stop telling yourself the painful stories that cause you to suffer.

Please know that you don't have to heal all areas of your life and psyche to become free from eating issues. However, you do have to be willing to take a critical look at those areas, tell yourself the truth about what's going on and begin to make changes if they're warranted. Even though our culture looks at an eating misalignment as something that can be fixed through diet and exercise alone, healing can never be complete unless it includes the spiritual perspective.

Ultimately, no longer relying on food to get happy means altering the underlying causes of your unhappiness and becoming more aligned with your spiritual nature. Because the truth about eating issues is that they aren't separate from your happiness. Any movement out of suffering that includes questioning misguided thinking and adjusting your lifestyle to support your happiness is also a movement toward becoming free from your eating issues. These things are inextricably linked.

The Truth About the Story of You and Food

Imagine that your life is a story. If food has been the center of your universe, the villain in your story, the ego—that negative chatterbox in your head who never seems to shut up—has been in charge of your eating and has most likely made your life a misery. The second character in your story is you. You are actually both the audience and the hero in your own story. Up until now, the conflict in your story has been caused by the two opposing desires created by the ego: the desire to experience taste pleasure and society's pressure to maintain a slim, sexy body. But now your story is taking a different turn.

We'll come back to the plot of your story and your heroic nature, but let's explore the ego's nature a bit more first. You may associate the term *ego* with someone who's conceited (someone who "has a big ego"). For our purposes, think of the ego as the fear-based, judgmental, lying voice in your head that makes you feel separate from other people. When you identify with this false persona that masquerades as you, you feel vulnerable and small, and don't trust other people. Why should you? If they're like you, they're out for themselves, and they could hurt you—or worse.

To stop identifying with the ego, you have to stop being fooled by its tricks. These are easier to recognize if we think of the ego as a character with three faces: the pleasure-seeking child, the critic and the dreamer.

The Pleasure-Seeking Child

Telling Yourself the Truth

This facet of the ego is the part of us that tempts us with the taste pleasure of junk food and turns a blind eye to the consequences of eating when we're not hungry or eating too much of the wrong foods. She is a trickster who deludes us by tempting us with a small sliver of truth: junk food tastes good. Defiantly, she ignores the rest of the truth: if we eat too much of it, we feel sick, bloated and drained. We might gain weight, feel upset with ourselves, and deprive our body of the nutrients it needs—a point that we often overlook.

When the child tempts us with pleasure food, she whispers things in our ears like, "Come on, just have a few bites. That can't hurt. You know you want to." Or "You've already blown your diet for the day, so what's the harm?" Or "You've worked so hard, you deserve a little pleasure." Her voice can be very compelling, and when we're under her influence, nothing matters except getting the food we crave into our chops right this minute.

Exercise: Getting Familiar with the Child Voice

Take out your journal and jot down some examples of what your child says to you. It's important to recognize the child voice instantly when she speaks in order to avoid going under her spell.

The Critic

Although the pleasure-seeking child rules when it comes to our tormented relationship with food, it's the nasty egoic villain called the critic who often dominates our relationship with our bodies. The voices are quite different, but the child and the critic are partners in crime, working together to make us miserable. The child tempts us with delicious junk food and if we give in and eat too much of it, we gain weight. Then, the critic steps in, making us feel guilty and shameful for overeating. The critic castigates us for not having the willpower to resist, dealing a wounding blow to our self-esteem.

Her message is that if only we could forgo the immediate gratification of pleasure food, we too could have perfectly shaped, slender bodies like the models and actors who grace magazine covers. Wagging her finger at us, she points to media images and says, "Why don't you look like that? If you weren't so spineless, you could have a body like that." She magnifies our every imperfection and sets the stage for villain number three, the dreamer.

The Dreamer

The dreamer serves as the silver lining in the critic's dark cloud. She tells us that if only we follow her advice and use an iron will to diet and exercise our way to a perfect body, we'll be home free. We'll lasso eternal happiness.

In the story of eating, weight and body-image misery, the plot goes like this: First, the pleasure-seeking child tempts you with pleasure food. Because it's hard to stop eating it, you inevitably overeat and gain weight. Then, the critic chastises you for this infraction, deflating your self-esteem and creating an even bigger opening for the child to return and offer immediate pleasure as a salve. You bounce back and forth between the two until you find yourself slumped over in a heap of mental, physical and emotional exhaustion.

Just when all seems lost, the dreamer appears, offering salvation. All of your past sins will be forgiven, the dreamer promises, if only you follow her advice. "It's simple," she says. "Just let me help you lose the weight, and your worries and suffering will be a thing of the past. Once you have a perfect body, you will conquer the world, and all of your dreams will come true."

Following the dreamer's advice, you dutifully stick to your diet, lose weight and find yourself looking and feeling fabulous. Even the critic has to bite her tongue. Because you're an emotional eater, to celebrate, you take yourself out for a decadent meal. Then, slowly but surely, you begin letting the pleasure-seeking child guide your eating again. After all, you've worked so hard that you deserve to get some pleasure now. A few pounds find their way back onto your frame. You feel upset with yourself for gaining weight and stuff down your sadness and remorse with pleasure food. More pounds pile on and pretty soon, you've put all your weight back on.

Our Hero: Essence

This is where the hero, the one who's aware of the villains' antics, takes over. Up to this point in the story, you innocently believed that you *were* the ego. It was perfectly reasonable for you to assume that the child, critic and dreamer were speaking with your own voice. Only now do you start to see that it's all been a ruse. You're not who you thought you were. Unbeknownst to you, you've been the hero all along.

Rather than this character you've been playing, a person with a name and personality, you are essence, the wise, mature, benevolent witness of both that character and the thought stream that constantly races through your consciousness. You could think of essence as the wise parent to the pleasure-seeking child, saying to her when she wants a cookie, "Not now, honey, maybe later." Or "You've had enough cookies. Eating more will make you feel bad, and it's not good for your body." Essence is the kind, gentle guide that corrals the child's impulses, counteracts the critic's harshness and sees through the dreamer's empty promises.

On an experiential level, essence is that place of inner calm and well-being that you tap into every day. Unless you meditate or do some other sort of practice designed to quiet your mind, you may not be aware of this place of inner calm. To experience essence right now, close your eyes and focus your attention on your hands. Get curious about the sensations there. Don't think about it. Just experience it.

Did you notice any tingling or a feeling of aliveness in your hands? That feeling is one of the manifestations of the subtle senses, and a clear indication that you are in essence.

So this is our story. In it, we're taking a journey that can't be measured in hours or miles, but that represents a huge leap in consciousness: moving out of the thinking mind, or egoic level of consciousness, and into pure awareness. The plot of the story and the spiritual evolutionary path for all human beings is seeing our true identity as essence and living from that place. This journey can also be described as moving out of your head and into your heart.

Meditation: Moving into Essence

Imagine a crystal-clear turquoise ocean. Feel the warmth of the sun on your skin. Now imagine yourself floating effortlessly in the waves. Feel yourself mesmerized by the rhythmic movement of the current. You are the embodiment of peace. No worries, no struggle. Just feel yourself effortlessly carried by the current, in the same way that life effortlessly carries you, directing you, supporting you in its wisdom. Allow yourself to feel the joy of simply being. Nothing needs to be added to you.

Feel the life that you are animating in this body that you are borrowing for the experience of humanness. Feel the liquid sunlight pouring over you, entering your skin. And as you focus your attention there, let yourself melt and merge with that sunlight. Let yourself relax out of physicality and merge with light. For a moment, let yourself release this character that you are playing at. Let go of all thoughts of the "me." Feel the vastness of this spiritual being that you are and have always been. You are nothing and everything simultaneously. You are radiant, spacious light.

All of the universes are contained within your being. There is no beginning and no end to you. You are ageless, deathless, formless, a divine presence. There is nothing that you are not and yet there is not an object you can point to and say, "That's me, there I am." You are the oneness from which all form emanates.

Suns and planets form and then they die and all the while, you remain unchanged, untouched by all of these occurrences. You are that which never comes and goes. You always remain this spacious, aware presence with no borders, no boundaries. Nothing can contain you.

Let yourself feel into the aliveness, feel the joy of being unbounded, of being completely free. What does that feel like? Know that this feeling sense of what you are, this spaciousness, is always available to you, in every moment. When you turn your attention away from thoughts and dive in between the thoughts, you disappear into this contented joy—this feeling of all is well, that what you are and what you have is enough.

The Truth About Thoughts

The simple truth about living with a human mind is that if you believe your stressful thoughts, the ones that come from the egoic mind, you will suffer. Yet ignoring thoughts is easier said than done because we're programmed from birth to pay attention to and believe our thoughts. When a stressful thought or a romantic thought about food pops into your head, the mind immediately produces reams of proof supporting that painful distillation of life or illusion about food.

But the truth about egoic thoughts is that you don't need them! They are fear-based, negative and untrue. Thoughts from the functional mind, however, are actually helpful. These enable you to balance your checkbook, formulate a strategic plan and keep your appointments. Obviously, you need your functional mind, but you can move happily and elegantly through life without the so-called help of your egoic thoughts.

Because you're programmed to believe that you *are* the thoughts running through your head, professing that you don't need your egoic thoughts is tantamount to heresy. Consequently, the only way to convince yourself that you don't need the egoic mind is to live without it and see what happens.

Start by paying attention to your thoughts. What are the thoughts that keep you riveted? Once you start keeping track of these, you will see that most of the thoughts that arise in your consciousness are circular, repetitive and stress-provoking. They keep you contracted and distracted, and they carefully omit the only guidance that could help to alleviate your suffering. Stop paying attention to and believing your stressful thoughts. This is easy to say and harder to do because, if you're like most people, you've reinforced the habit of listening to your stressful thoughts over many years. The way to ignore them is to see, over and over again, that they never tell the whole truth. Although they may contain a kernel of truth, which is what hooks you, overall they present a distorted, unpleasant story. When you see the truth about stressful thoughts and commit yourself to ignoring them, the ego will be out of a job.

Once you start paying attention to your thoughts, you'll notice that they weave themselves into stories that relate to judging, evaluating, analyzing and characterizing based on only one criterion: How does this situation impact me?

That question will naturally lead to others: Is this situation good for me or do I need to take action to protect myself? How can I manipulate life and people to get what I want? How can I maximize my pleasure and minimize my pain?

If you see yourself as a "me," as a mere body subject to illness, injury and death, naturally, you will live in fear. The Indian sage Nisargadatta Maharaj, whose teachings form the foundation of this book, said, "Don't you see that all your problems are your body's problems—food, clothing, shelter, family, friends, name, fame, security, survival—all these lose their meaning the moment you realize that you may not be a mere body."

The "me," or ego, is not even a thing, per se. It's the belief that you are a body, separate from all other human beings, that needs protecting. From this belief, it follows that if you don't take care of this body and make sure it has what it needs to survive and be happy, other bodies will move in and snatch up all of the planet's limited resources. You won't get what you need and you will be annihilated.

Telling Yourself the Truth

The belief that you are separate stirs up fears and keeps you feeling vulnerable and off balance. This is the ego in problem-generator mode. Because life never fulfills all of your desires by delivering all pleasure and no pain, when life doesn't conform to your preferences, the ego leads you to believe that you have problems. Then, it comes to the rescue by formulating plans to solve those problems and keep you safe. Whenever you notice that you feel on edge, stressed or afraid, you can bet that you bought into one of the ego's problematic thoughts.

Yet living *without* the egoic mind's guidance moves you into a different world, where stress and contraction are transformed into peace, easefulness and boundless freedom. You connect with life directly through your senses rather than through the veil of thoughts and feelings. In this way, you have an experience of essence, and you realize that there is something much wiser moving inside you that has been guiding your life all along. When you surrender to this truly wise guidance, which comes in the form of intuitions and insights rather than thoughts, and stop paying attention to your egoic thoughts, your life becomes much happier.

The Truth About Romanticizing Food

If you believe your romantic thoughts about food, the ones that convince you that food has the power to entertain, comfort or distract you from your emotions, eventually you will follow them to the refrigerator, and you will have a challenging time maintaining a healthy weight. Romanticizing food means fantasizing about it, imbuing it with qualities and powers that it doesn't possess, or fixating on the pleasurable aspect of eating it. When you imagine that food has anything to offer you other than nice-tasting nutrition, you can find yourself eating for the wrong reasons and gaining weight. If you're eating solely for pleasure rather than nutrition, eating emotionally, entertaining yourself with food or imagining how food will taste, you're romanticizing it. But the truth is that food *can't* give you unending pleasure, make you happy when you're sad, comfort you when you're lonely, relieve your stress, revive you when you feel tired or reignite your joie de vivre when you feel listless or bored.

When you romanticize chocolate chip cookies, eating them distracts you for a few moments, and then leaves you with the situation and feeling that led you to reach for them in the first place, along with a feeling of disappointment in yourself for giving in to temptation. You know that it isn't the best choice, yet you go for it anyway. Why? Because even though you've been conditioned to see the behavior as weakness, on a certain level, eating the cookies is a based in a loving impulse to shield yourself from discomfort. It's an innocent gesture to self-soothe that has been your habit.

Telling Yourself the Truth

You don't court chocolate chip cookies by sending them flowers or romantic cards, but that doesn't stop you from romanticizing them by lusting after them in your mind. Consciously, you know that food can't curl up with you at night and make you feel loved, but somewhere deep down you believe that it is your most coveted source of pleasure.

If you're in the habit of romanticizing food, you're probably used to asking yourself:

What do I want to eat? What am I in the mood for?
    or
What taste would I like to have in my mouth?
    rather than

What nutrition could my body use?

Romanticizing food is a way of deluding yourself by playing *Let's Pretend*. "Let's pretend that I can change my unpleasant experience into a pleasant one through food." It's magical thinking that only tells part of the truth and leaves out the bloating, shame, guilt, listlessness, ill health and possible weight gain that come with eating too much comfort food. It's like picking up a coin, believing that you can peel the heads side away from the tails side and put only that one side in your pocket. The truth is that you can't peel the pleasure away from the pain.

Ultimately, healing your relationship with food is about withdrawing your romantic projections from it. When you do this, you are able to see the whole truth—that food is a source of pain as well as pleasure when used in ways that it was never intended. If you form a new habit of seeing food's primary function as meeting the nutritional needs of the body rather than seeing it as comfort, entertainment or distraction, you'll stop suffering over it. The reward for this shift in your relationship with food is a healthier, slimmer body that is yours to keep for the rest of your life, without worry or struggle.

The Truth About a Partial Truth

A partial truth is not a truth, although it's easy to delude ourselves into thinking that it is. The mind hooks us with a thin sliver of truth (usually a negative or distorted perception) about something in life and asks us to believe that this sliver is the whole truth. For example, since childhood I've had a tendency to lose things. My ego hooks me with this small truth about myself with the intention of creating a negative feeling. It tries to convince me that the whole truth about me is contained in this one trait: I'm a person who loses things and that's a bad thing and therefore I'm an inadequate person. But the ego leaves out the rest of the story. The whole truth about my character is that it includes many other positive qualities that round out the entirety of who I am.

It's only when we forget the whole picture of who we are and buy into the ego's small truth that we suffer. Forming a painful, myopic view is what the ego does best. If a thought causes you to feel bad, you can know that it's too small a sliver to really be true, and that there's no need for you to waste your time by giving it your attention.

The sliver of truth about food is that it tastes good. There's no problem with this except that it leaves out the rest of the truth: if you eat too much or consistently eat unhealthy food, you experience a slew of negative consequences. In exchange for the few moments of pleasure you enjoy while overeating your favorite food, you experience much longer-term discomfort. From essence, the wise part of ourselves, we see the whole truth of this lousy bargain. We may occasionally still indulge, but from a place of awareness and conscious choice.

Food Freedom And Truth

There's a world of difference between this place and the self-deluded place of the ego that plays the *Let's Pretend* game. From this place of clear seeing, we can form a new, healthy relationship with food—one that includes the pleasure of eating because it's part of the whole truth.

Exercise: The Whole Truth About Food

In the table below or in your journal, list the costs and benefits of eating too much or eating the wrong things when you're not hungry. Some of the costs might be negative feelings such as shame, blame, self-castigation, regret, anger or sadness, not to mention damaged self-esteem, indigestion, listlessness and potential weight gain.

This exercise helps us to see the whole truth of our behavior all at once. It raises the question: Am I really willing to accept all of the consequences of this behavior? If we can get into the habit of seeing the whole truth of our behavior, we'll be less likely to follow the pleasure-seeking child when she tempts us.

Benefits	Costs
1. A nice taste in the mouth	1. Taste pleasure is fleeting
2.	2. Possible weight gain
3.	3. Shame
	4. Low self-esteem
	5. Ill health
	6. No appetite for healthy food

The Truth About Loving Food

The truth about loving food is that it can never love us back. Food is just food. It's fuel that gives the body energy to go about its business—working, playing, thinking, talking and performing the functions of the autonomic nervous system. In spite of its primary function as fuel, food is not repulsive medicine that you have to hold your nose to choke down. The fact that even healthy food tastes good and is pleasurable to eat is an undeniable part of the eating equation.

With so many other sensory pleasures available, why have so many of us become fixated on and addicted to food? What's its allure? People who've spent countless waking hours thinking about and anticipating their next meal would swear that food is their favorite thing in the universe and that eating trumps all other worldly pleasures. And many would say that it captures our hearts and imaginations because it looks, smells and tastes so good. It appeals to all five of our senses. From the moment we place a forkful in our mouths, there's no denying the pleasure it gives us.

If you're nodding away at that notion, then answer this question: When was the last time you *just ate* while you were eating? When was the last time you ate without watching television, listening to the radio, reading, driving or having a conversation? When, of your own volition, did you just eat without coupling it with another experience?

If you can't remember the last time you just ate, how does the idea sound to you? Imagine eating your favorite food all by yourself with no other distractions. Does that sound appealing? If not, why not? If food were truly the love of your life, why would you need to pair eating with another activity? Why wouldn't that incredibly pleasurable experience be enough? Is it possible that your idea of eating doesn't match up to the truth about it? If so, perhaps you haven't been seeing the whole truth of food.

There's no denying that while food is in our mouths, it tastes good. Yet prolonging the pleasurable sensation requires inserting more and more food. And if we do that, we all know what happens. We overfill our stomachs, and after a short while, the enjoyment of eating shifts into something else. The pleasure turns into pain. The anticipation turns into aversion.

This is the inseparable nature of pairs of opposites. Hindu and Buddhist philosophies teach that the pleasures of the physical dimension are transient and, if not taken in moderation, bear within them the seeds of commensurate pain. The truth about loving food is that the good taste lasts for only a short while and if we try to draw out the taste pleasure, our love turns to hate.

Knowing this, does it really make sense to love food? Is it rational to love an experience so passionately when its pleasurable nature is so fleeting? Does it make sense to idolize an experience that so quickly becomes unpleasant? Are there other ways we can take care of ourselves that are truly fulfilling and nurturing? Ask yourself, "How can I feed my soul and experience the kind of joy that can't fade or turn into its opposite?"

Merging with Emotions

Whenever we feel a negative emotion, the person next to us doesn't feel it, so there's a tendency to think that the emotion belongs to us alone. We take ownership of it. The problem with taking ownership of an emotion, rather than seeing it as just a neutral phenomenon arising in consciousness, is that owning it makes it much easier to identify with. When you identify with an emotion, it's like you actually *become* the feeling. But the truth about emotions is that even though they erupt in our body, they don't belong to us.

Illustration of a Person Merged with an Emotion

Illustration of a Person Disidentified with an Emotion

We also tend to think that emotions provide us with important information that we need to act upon immediately. But no matter what we may have been told, emotions don't provide trustworthy guidance for how to navigate our lives or relationships. They don't provide confirmation that we have the correct take on a situation and that the other guy is all wet. And they don't justify bad behavior. Just because we feel angry doesn't make it okay for us to express it in a way that blames or punishes someone else. Contrary to popular belief, talking about a circumstance that triggered anger, unless it comes from a balanced, dispassionate place, often exacerbates it.

Food Freedom And Truth

Yet there is wisdom in how life works—because negative emotions do serve an important purpose. Like everything else in life, emotions happen *for you*, not to you. You are not their victim. Ideally, they function as alarm clocks, waking you up to the fact that you just believed an untrue thought. When an emotion hits, there's no going back. As hard as you may try, you can't "unfeel" it. Your choices are to try to avoid feeling it through an addictive substance or behavior, express it to others with an agenda of trying to make them responsible for it, or welcome it, allow it to be there, and question the underlying thought that gave birth to it.

People in the throes of a negative emotion often later say things like, "I have no idea what just got into me. Forgive me, I wasn't myself." And that's the truth. When a negative emotion erupts, it's like being possessed by a negative alter ego. And once we identify with a negative emotion, things go from bad to worse. Our tendency is to blow it up even more by inventing plenty of reasons to justify it.

Being caught up in an emotion is like being caught in a thunderstorm without an umbrella. Your emotional sky was clear and, all of a sudden, you're soaked. Your body feels contracted and contorted and you're frantically looking for a safe, dry place—a way to get out of the storm and back to the previous moment, when life felt good.

But if you realize that emotions, like thunderstorms, pass, you can relax. Thankfully, everything that arises, including emotions, eventually subsides and causes no harm. The thunderstorm can't hurt the sky and emotions can't hurt you. After a thunderstorm passes, it's as if it never happened. The sky is left unchanged.

Telling Yourself the Truth

Positive emotions, such as joy and happiness, are no more real than negative emotions. They're just aspects of who we are naturally, aspects of essence, and we freely experience them anytime we're not in the contraction of a negative emotion.

All that said, persistent sadness or depression can be an indication that your life is out of balance. While emotions show you that your conditioning has been triggered, it's important to look at whether you need to change your outer circumstances as well as doing your inner work.

There are two important truths to know about negative emotions: 1) although they don't feel good when they hit, they're tolerable and don't stay long and 2) they always come bearing gifts. Wisely, life ensures that emotions create strong sensations in your body to wake you up to a new opportunity to free yourself from the bondage of conditioning. Emotions are signs that you are ready to see through and release an erroneous belief that has cost you precious aliveness. If we are present and understand these essential truths about emotions, we can use them to propel us more deeply into the freedom that is our birthright.

Exercise: Allowing Yourself to Feel an Emotion

The next time a strong emotion arises, find a place to be alone for a few minutes. Close your eyes and allow yourself to feel it.

What is present now?
Can you get in touch with that _____ and just allow it to be present?
Can you actually welcome it?
Where do you feel it in your body?
What is the sensation?
If it had a color, what color would it be?
What shape is it?
What texture?
What size?

Be sure not to feed the feeling with more thoughts and stories. Just allow it to be present without any agenda for it to go away.

Is it still okay for it to be there?
If it had a voice, what would it say?
Periodically, ask what is happening with the _____ that you now think of as a [fuzzy red ball or black cylinder].

The Truth About Hunger

Few other words in the English language evoke more fear and resistance than *hunger*. We're used to seeing it flanked by equally scary words like *pestilence, famine, disease, starvation* and *death*. And hunger avoidance is built into many cultures and religions. In Judaism, people wish each other well by praying that their children will never know hunger. In most societies, ascending the socioeconomic ladder and landing in the cushy land of wealth and prosperity has meant transcending this ancient hallmark of life. Yet in the West, much of the population has sacrificed health for the idea that hunger is a bad thing.

I'll let you in on a little secret: The ego is always seeking comfort. Any prospect of discomfort, no matter how small, sends it scurrying for the exit. Hunger is no exception. The ego says, "Why should I have to experience the discomfort of hunger if I don't have to? I know life will throw me a lot of curveballs, but hunger doesn't need to be one of them. I can feed the hunger monster anytime I want, and at least avoid that one discomfort."

But have you ever considered that hunger might be an integral part of the optimal functioning of the body? Like eating, resting and exercising, perhaps bodies need to experience hunger to run well. Could it be that hunger is one natural way the body helps us maintain a healthy size?

Now forget health for a moment. Have you ever noticed how delicious food tastes when you're hungry? Even a carrot tastes like manna from heaven. When you allow yourself to get tummy-rumbling hungry, you enjoy your food in a way that isn't possible when your tank is still full. When you're not hungry, the taste of food and the experience of eating are not nearly as satisfying.

The truth is that hunger is a necessary part of the equation if our goal is to have our bodies maintain a healthy weight. But how do we deal with our fear and resistance toward it? Before we dive in, let me clarify: I'm not talking about hunger so great that you feel like a ravenous, crazed maniac capable of cannibalizing your next-door neighbor. I'm talking about hunger that manifests as that slightly uncomfortable, tummy-rumbling sensation you experience when your stomach is empty.

The first step to overcoming this fear is to unearth the meanings you've given to hunger. What are the stories you tell yourself about it? What are the beliefs and concepts you have that cause you to recoil from it and reach frantically for anything edible at the first sign of it?

Here are a few beliefs I've come across in my travels:

1. If I let myself get hungry, my blood sugar will drop. I'll get shaky and I won't be able to function.

2. If I let myself get hungry, I'll eat everything in sight. I won't be able to stop.

3. Hunger is too uncomfortable. I won't be able to bear it.

4. It's too scary. I can't let myself go there. If I get hungry, I'll get more and more uncomfortable until it becomes unbearable.

Let's take a closer look at each of these notions:

1. If I let myself get hungry, my blood sugar will drop. I'll get shaky and I won't be able to function. This fear is the result of a misunderstanding. Again, I'm not suggesting that you live with hunger for hours and hours or experience some extreme version of it that impacts your energy level or blood sugar. I'm suggesting that you open yourself up to a natural sensation that cues you when your body is ready for you to eat a meal.

2. If I let myself get hungry, I'll eat everything in sight. I won't be able to stop. "I'll eat everything in sight" is just a story we told ourselves to keep from seeing the real truth of hunger. Although it may be true that in the past, you've let yourself get very hungry and then used the sensation as an excuse to justify overeating, regular hunger and overeating don't have to go together.

3. Hunger is too uncomfortable. I won't be able to bear it. Is that really true? When you say that, you are imagining a scary future and tying that to your concept of hunger. I challenge you to let go of your assumption, allow yourself to get hungry and see what happens. See if you're telling yourself a fib or not.

4. It's too scary. I can't let myself go there. If I get hungry, I'll get more and more uncomfortable until it becomes unbearable. Ask yourself, "What am I afraid of?" Is it starvation? Is it discomfort? What is so frightening about letting yourself experience hunger? Write these fears down and take a risk. Allow yourself to get hungry and see if your fears are realized.

Hunger Exercise

Now it's your turn. Try letting yourself get hungry before you eat. Each time you're about to eat something, ask yourself, "Am I hungry?" If the answer is no, wait until you get a yes before lifting your fork to your lips. See what happens. Give yourself the chance to experience hunger as it is, free from your concepts about it. See the whole truth of it, rather than living according to your uninvestigated ideas about it.

I've personally learned to like the feeling of being light and feeling hungry. I like the way food tastes when I've let myself get hungry before I dig in. I especially like the result of being hungry at times: being thin and feeling energetic and light on my feet.

I've gotten into the habit of being hungry some of the time, so it's not a problem. Part of what has helped me to not view feeling hungry as a problem is that it has become a habit, a normal part of my everyday experience. It's also no longer a problem if I can't eat when I'm hungry. I know I'll get around to eating eventually. All the fear around it is gone. Because I trust that I will be able to eat at some point, I don't have to manage the feeling in my stomach by constantly checking in on it.

The Truth About What You're Eating

People asking for help to heal their food misalignment often say things like "I'm so tired of suffering. Just tell me what to do, and I'll do it." But when I encourage them to eat differently and give up junk food that has no nutritional value, they make a beeline for the door. "I'll do anything you want, but don't ask me to give up the food I love," they say.

After a few weeks, they'll tell me that they've been vigilant about bringing more awareness to their eating, that they've been making sure their tummies are rumbling before they eat, resting, feeding their souls and speaking their truths—all of which are integral to healing. But they often leave out the food component, and no one can leave out the food component and expect to heal this issue. No one can continue to eat the same foods, not monitor portion size, or eat when they're not hungry and expect to achieve and maintain a natural, healthy body size.

Sure, it's nice to imagine that you can take off the weight and eat whatever you want, but it doesn't work that way. I'm not saying that you can't ever treat yourself with food. You don't have to be perfect. I'm far from perfect, but it doesn't impact my health or weight, so I don't worry about it. That being said, it took a few years of strictly following the principles of good eating before I felt comfortable getting looser. Until you reach that point of normalizing your relationship with food, and are no longer romanticizing it, it's best to be strict with yourself.

Trying to be moderate about eating just doesn't work for people with a history of food-related issues. And the food industry certainly isn't interested in helping. It's well known in the industry that creating foods with the right balance of fat, sugar and salt makes them hard to resist. A chocolate chip cookie is a perfect example. Such foods are *designed* to be irresistible. The food conglomerates' profits depend on making you believe that their products are the earthly equivalent to heaven in your mouth. Who needs an apple when you can have an apple pie pocket?

If we all woke up tomorrow morning and decided to consume calories from whole foods (edibles that are grown rather than made), food manufacturers would be in big trouble. Even with their state-of-the-art labs and legions of food scientists, they haven't been able to figure out how to make bananas or broccoli or brown rice. Consequently, to create products that they can charge a premium for, they have to process real food and turn it into something else: junk.

Think about it. Food companies are in business to make money, not to keep us healthy. They maximize profits by:

1. Keeping food costs low. To do this, they increase crop yields by:
   a. Using fertilizers made from petrochemicals.
   b. Spraying crops with poisonous pesticides.
2. Creating a market of loyal customers, preferably addicts. The companies have engineered food that is irresistible by adding lots of sugar, high-fructose corn syrup, salt and fat. Consequently, we have become addicted to these overblown tastes. There is no more stable market than a customer base full of addicts.
3. Brainwashing us into buying nutrient-bereft junk with advertising that stresses taste and low prices.

Telling Yourself the Truth

Taste buds are creatures of habit. As our most malleable body parts, they can easily be coaxed into loving almost anything. But even though they've become addicted to the overblown taste of junk, we can train them to love healthy food the same way we trained them to love the junk. Here's how: First, trade in your junk food habit for a healthy food habit by buying fresh produce, whole grains and proteins at the supermarket. Then, commit to a habit of eating healthy food day after day. Habits are formed by repetition. Before long, healthy food will start to taste amazing, better than the junk ever did.

Contrary to what you might believe, creating a healthy relationship with food *doesn't* mean sacrificing taste. You don't eliminate the pleasure of eating, *you simply eliminate eating solely for pleasure,* and that's a big difference. Healthy food has a wholesome, clean taste that's satisfying in a way that junk can never be. When you eat healthy, you are rewarded with a more energetic, younger-looking and better-feeling body. You also get the pleasure of great taste and the pride of knowing that you are treating your body (and the planet) well and doing your part to ensure its future health and well-being.

Food Freedom And Truth

Meditation for Wise Food Choices

Sit comfortably in a place where you can be alone for 10 or 15 minutes. Become aware of the movement of your breathing. Allow any worries or tensions of the day to slip away. It's as if they are miles and miles away. Take another deep breath. Fill your lungs to capacity, hold the breath in for a moment, and now slowly exhale. Allow any stress to leave your body as you exhale.

Other thoughts may arise. Just notice them passing like clouds drifting by in the sky of your mind. Allow your eyes and face to soften and relax. Just let any lines of tension release. You are becoming more and more at peace, more and more relaxed, as if you are floating on a fluffy, white cloud of peace. Float and drift. Take another deep breath through your nose and exhale completely out of your mouth. Allow any remaining tension to leave with your breath.

With every breath, become more and more and relaxed. Relax your forehead and scalp. Just let those muscles relax. Let your whole face relax. Feel the tension release in your shoulders and back. Feel the tensions drain away from your body, leaving your shoulders, arms and hands, and radiating out your fingertips. It feels so good to give yourself this gift of relaxation and peace.

Now, imagine yourself in front of banquet table arrayed with junk food, foods that are poisonous, that are harmful to your body. They are the fattening, empty calories that you used to eat and caused your overweight. Imagine yourself pushing these foods away. Push them off of the table. You reject these foods because you have made a decision to love yourself and your body. You have decided to live your life in a slender, energetic, healthy, fit body. You have no use for empty-calorie, life-draining foods that cause ill health, bloating and weight gain.

Now, imagine filling this table with healthy, life-giving foods. Fruits, vegetables, whole foods and pure, clean water. Imagine eating these nourishing, healthy foods and enjoying every bite. Your new eating habits feel so good to you, so natural. You feel so pure and light. Imagine seeing yourself drinking lots of pure, clean water. You remember to eat only when your body is physically hungry, when you feel some tummy rumbling that lets you know that your tummy is empty.

You are more motivated now than ever before because the reward of being healthier is so appealing to you. Now you know in your heart that you can achieve the healthy body that you have always wanted. As each day passes, you find that you have increased feelings of confidence and self-esteem. As you move closer to your healthier weight, the realization that you can become a healthier, more energetic person makes you feel happy and so proud of yourself.

Feel an overwhelming sense of confidence and security rising up within you as you realize that you have taken control of your life. You no longer have to listen to and follow the dictates of the pleasure-seeking child. To your delight, your taste for food is changing and high-calorie, low-nutrition foods no longer pull you in the same

THE TRUTH ABOUT DESIRE

Desire

To understand the truth about eating issues, we need to understand desire. We suffer over our desires because we can only desire what we don't have—and that hurts. However, desires also fuel our actions and bring us the experiences we need to grow. Without them, life on the physical plane would come to a grinding halt.

Yet at a certain point in our evolution, we become wise to the nature of desire and see that following it blindly brings unhappiness. When this happens, we have the option to choose not to follow our desires and instead grow consciously without suffering.

A desire comes into being when we identify with the thought "I want." It's possible for that thought to arise and subside without ceremony or discomfort. But when we focus on it and give it our attention, there is a merging. On some level, we come to believe that we *are* this thought. If I want ice cream when I can't have it and I persist in following the thought "I want ice cream," I merge with it. By fixating on it, I become this desire and suffer.

Identification with painful thoughts like "I want" is the root of all human suffering: it's the only thing that has the power to keep us from our natural happiness. Take a moment to really let that set in—because it's the key to waking up out of your ego. Learning how to not identify with desires is how you transcend and shift out of the false self, become free, and open yourself to enjoying life from the natural peace and joy of your true self.

Addiction: The Ego's Answer to What It Doesn't Like

When it comes right down to it, there isn't much the ego likes about life because life almost never shows up exactly the way the ego wants it to. In those rare moments when life feels perfect, the ego frets about losing that experience. It scares itself into imagining a future bereft of those perfect conditions. In other words, being a human being provides no safe, happy sanctuary for the ego. Life generally doesn't feel as good as the dreamer's fantasies, so the ego looks to swap its experience of the present moment for another moment that it imagines will feel better.

Often, addiction serves as the ego's answer to what it doesn't like about life, with the other, better moment consisting of an immediate pleasure hit from food, shopping, alcohol, drugs, gambling or sex. For food addicts, this may play out in very simple ways: we're paying bills or doing some other task we find boring and then unconsciously traipse to the refrigerator.

Our physical world is governed by physical laws, but also by laws of duality. Wherever you find pleasure, pain is sure to follow. In the same way that it is physically impossible to separate two sides of a coin, it is impossible to separate pairs of opposites. But the ego imagines that it can transcend duality and lasso only the pleasure and none of the pain of addictive behaviors or substances, and it tricks us into believing this as well. It hooks us with a memory of how wonderful a hot fudge sundae tastes and, all of a sudden, we hop in the car and speed to the ice cream store, carefully avoiding thoughts about the negative consequences of our choice.

We desperately want to believe that we can bend life to our will and experience only its pleasures. Many of our fantasies are about just that, which is why they're called fantasies. They exist only in the realm of our imaginations. When we turn to food to distract us from emotional pain, we are deluding ourselves into believing that we can experience only the pleasurable aspect of eating, without the pain.

The next time you sense an urge to change your experience of life by eating, ask yourself, "What is it that I'm trying to avoid through food? What experience am I trying not to have? What am I resisting?" Ask yourself if reaching for food will satisfy you forever or enable you to permanently dodge whatever you're trying to avoid through taste pleasure. Then ask yourself, "Is there something here that is enjoying even the experience I'm trying to change? Is there something here that's delighting in this experience that I call distasteful?"

How to Stop Creating Desire

Desires are created when you place your attention on the thought "I want." When you fixate on "I want," whether it's a call from your new lover or a hot fudge sundae, you create a desire for the pleasure you imagine that experience will bring you. You fondly remember the past pleasure that you enjoyed with that person or food and project an expectation to experience it again.

Yet that memory is a story about what happened rather than what actually happened. It's a romanticization rather than the truth of the event. You romanticize the other person by remembering only his good qualities and the fun you had with him, rather than his chronic lateness or overspending. In other words, you leave out the totality of his humanness. You romanticize the hot fudge sundae by thinking only about how good the last one tasted while ignoring any unpleasant side effects you might have experienced after you ate it, such as a bloated belly, regret or difficulty putting on your jeans the next day. Creating the story of desire requires a narrowing of the aperture of our seeing. This is self-delusion. Because it leaves out so much of the truth, desire is always based on a lie.

You can stop creating desire by no longer buying into the thought "I want" and by realizing that it is based on a delusional belief that you can pick and choose the part of the truth you want to experience. You want to experience the party in your mouth that the hot fudge sundae delivers, but you can't separate that experience from the truth that the sundae contains hundreds of empty calories.

The Truth about Desire

Here's an example of how this works: I was in England visiting family and I wanted to eat the baked tortilla chips that I was used to getting back home. After some investigation, I discovered that English supermarkets didn't carry baked tortilla chips. Did I keep pining for these chips after my disappointing discovery that it wasn't possible to procure them? No. Very soon, I stopped thinking about them and, consequently, stopped wanting them. The rational, pragmatic part of me took over. It realized that it's pointless to desire a food when there's no possibility of fulfilling that desire.

Thinking is everything! It's the key to disempowering our cravings and the key to our entire experience of life. Without thoughts about food, we have no food issues, and without food issues, we have no weight problem. How do you stop wanting the addictive food that you've been telling yourself you have to have? Simple. You stop eating it.

If you want to stop creating a desire that keeps you suffering, when the thought "I want" arises, recognize that it's a story that doesn't tell the whole truth. This awareness alone will dramatically reduce its power. Then, don't feed the desire with more thoughts or stories about how wonderful it will be to obtain the particular object. Adding more lines to the story just causes the desire to get bigger by making it seem even more compelling. This makes you feel even more justified in wanting what you want. Notice the thoughts, realize the lie they represent, and turn away from them. Choose to do or think about something else instead.

Exercise: The Freedom in Giving Something Up

To test the premise from this section—that you have to give something up for good to stop wanting it—pick a food that you feel out of control around that has little or no nutritional value. Decide to give up this food permanently. To help strengthen your resolve, decide that this item is no longer food to you. This really is true because if it doesn't have nutritional value, it's not food. Resolve that it's gone from your life for good, not just for a week or a month or two, but gone. Then, notice what happens to your desire for it. For a few days, you may still think about it. But once the pleasure-seeking child realizes that tempting you with this food isn't going to work, she gives up, and thoughts about that food will no longer arise.

How to Stop Suffering over Desires

Whether we like it or not, desires are a part of life. Nearly everything we do is driven by them. Our stomach growls, the desire to eat something arises, and we walk to the refrigerator. Our car's gas tank reads empty, the desire to ride rather than push the car home arises, and we pull into a gas station. As human beings, we may never be entirely free of desires, but we can make our relationship with them hurt less by not needing them to be met.

The basis of desire is an assumption that we're missing something, that if only we can get that thing, we'll be satisfied and happy. This leaves us with an uncomfortable sense of longing that we attempt to alleviate by trying to obtain the object of our desire. After all, if we believe that we need to get what we want in order to be happy, whenever we don't get it, we suffer. But if we can simply notice a desire arising, there's no problem. We won't suffer over it. Realizing that desires can arise and that we don't have to follow them or achieve them is a great epiphany. It means that wisdom has bloomed in our consciousness, creating the possibility of a new, happier life.

How do we reach this genuine understanding and not just pay it lip service when the habit of following desires is so deeply entrenched in us? We can start by forming the habit of moving into essence by asking, "Is there something here right now that is already full, complete and at peace? Is there something that is enjoying this moment, just the way it is?" Asking these questions automatically moves us out of the ego and into the silent, aware presence that lies at the heart of who we really are. When we're aligned with the ego, we want something. We believe that we aren't enough and don't have enough or, even if we are enough and have enough right now, we still fret, because we'll surely be lacking in the future. When we're aligned with essence, we're at peace in the knowledge that we have everything we need.

Sometimes, a desire feels so compelling that we convince ourselves we're powerless to resist it. As soon as we identify, or merge, with this thought, the mechanism of believing that we need the object of our desire in order to be happy turns us into desire embodied. Then, it literally feels like we'll die if we don't get what we want.

Understanding that we're all programmed to follow desires and suffer over them can help you feel compassionate toward yourself when you fall into this trap. To stop suffering over a desire, debunk the underlying assumption that holds it in place. Remember to ask yourself if you really want the whole picture of what following your desire will bring, rather than just the thin sliver of truth about it that the ego is peddling. Recognize that desire is a natural part of life and that just because a desire appears in your consciousness doesn't mean you have to follow it. If you don't follow it, it can't hook you and you won't suffer over it. If you recognize desire as merely the thought "I want," a thought that arises and subsides like all other thoughts, and don't give it any importance by identifying with it, you thwart the "desire equals suffering" equation.

The Truth about Desire

Who Is the "I" Who Wants?

When a desire such as "I want to lose weight so I can attract the attention of potential lovers" or "I want to eat a whole package of cookies right now" arises, who is the "I" that wants? Is it essence? Or is it the ego?

The next time a desire arises and you have a compelling urge to fill it, close your eyes and ask yourself, "Who is this 'I'?" See if you can find it. Resist the tendency to rush to come up with an answer, although that's exactly what the ego will want to do to avoid the discomfort of not knowing. Try to just allow yourself to not know, to live in the question, in the space of humility that opens up as a result of your willingness to live in the unknown. As you rest in the quiet, allow the original desire to melt away. When that happens, you'll find yourself in a familiar place, one that you've visited many times before. You go there when you daydream or when you first wake up in the morning in that not-quite-asleep, not-quite-awake state. You experience it when you forget yourself for a moment, looking at natural beauty, an animal or a baby.

Shifting into essence feels familiar because it is your natural state—your true home. It is so satisfying to hang out there because it is the direct experience of "all is well." As soon as you shift into essence, no false story of identifying with anything or as anyone can survive. From this place there is no "me" left to experience anything. Without the "I" thought dancing around in your head, the contrived barrier of ego that has been mediating between you and experience disappears, and you realize that, in spite of what you have been conditioned to believe, you are not this "I" and never have been this "I." You see that you are instead the awareness in which this "I" arises. This realization can bring huge relief.

When you step back into awareness, you realize you are *that which is aware of both the "I" and the thought.* So when a thought such as "Boy, that chocolate cake looks good. I really want a slice" arises, you are able to disempower the craving and separate from it. Alternatively, when you believe that the "I" that wants is the totality of who you are, and life doesn't deliver what you want in a given moment, you suffer. You identify and merge with this "I" and think that you are it.

The process of disidentification is totally logical: it just requires that you remind yourself that you can't be the "I" who wants because you are the one who is noticing it. You are that which is aware of desire because you are reporting that it exists. When you think you *are* an object or a belief or a desire, it's because, unwittingly, you've identified with it and given it power. This is easily demonstrated whenever people's pet beliefs are challenged. You can be engaged in a pleasant conversation with someone when, all of a sudden, their hackles go up. All you did was disagree with their belief, but, because they've identified with that belief, they feel personally attacked. From their perspective, it actually feels as if you're trying to take their life from them.

That said, I absolutely do not recommend pointing this out to others with comments such as "Hey, you just got defensive because you are identified with that belief of yours. I challenged the belief. I didn't attack you." If you say something like that, it's likely that the other person, who is already feeling contracted and identified with her ego, will interpret it as an attack, an attempt to make her wrong. This will likely drive her even more deeply into her ego.

The Truth about Desire

The "I" who wants is the ego, of course, because desire generation is one of the ego's most important functions. Our true self doesn't want or need anything. Why would it? It is everything already. It's pointless to ask, "What does essence, which embodies everything already, want?"

Desire Versus Intention

There are two kinds of desire: those that come from essence, which we'll call *intentions*, and those that come from the ego. Intentions that come from essence are aligned with fulfilling your life purpose. For example, if part of your life purpose includes becoming a musician, you will want to learn how to play a musical instrument. These kinds of intentions don't produce suffering. Following them is simply following a true movement within you, and that feels good.

Desires that come from the ego are a different thing altogether. These can cause intense suffering because they're often rooted in the intention to be separate by becoming superior and admired. Wanting to be above or better than other people moves us away from them and, ultimately, away from love, which is what we really are. In wanting to be above the crowd, we create a wall that isolates us and keeps us disconnected. Our worldview becomes "us versus them," and we move further and further away from love toward a lonely and painful existence.

The dreamer is the egoic character that we identify with when we want to lose weight to look "hot" and turn heads. More than anything, the dreamer wants to be admired, to be special, and she spins the story that admiration will bring fulfillment and lasting happiness. But when we lose weight and attract more attention from others, is it true that the attention brings complete and perfect happiness that lasts forever?

If you've attained your ideal weight at some point in your life, did the dreamer's promise come true? Did the attention bring complete and perfect everlasting happiness? Were there downsides to the attention? Did the increased attention bring any added worry or stress?

What about the desire to experience taste pleasure? Here, the ego as pleasure-seeking child tempts you by getting you to crave certain foods. She coaxes you into imagining how much you would enjoy the taste of them. If you're not feeling great, you may imagine that eating certain foods will make you feel better. That's because the ego is rarely satisfied with life as it unfolds and demands an experience of happiness in every moment. When life doesn't deliver, it goes searching for a pleasure fix and creates desire. The child says, "I want to feel good now and a hot fudge sundae will do the trick." She retrieves a memory of how a hot fudge sundae tastes and says, "Yep, that's what I'm talking about. That's what I want."

If you indulge that desire, you feel satisfied for a moment, not so much because of the experience of eating the sundae, although it provides a few fleeting seconds of taste enjoyment, but because you're no longer tormented by the unfulfilled desire. It's the *cessation of the desire* that brings the feeling of relief, not the sundae.

Egoic desires bring suffering, so when they end, we feel happy again. But then we're left with the consequences of our action, the guilt and remorse we feel for doing something that we really didn't want to do. We feel disappointed in ourselves and that generally lasts longer than the two minutes we spent eating the hot fudge sundae.

The next time you're in the throes of an egoic desire, try to remember that egoic desires are all trumped up and ultimately don't deliver the happiness they promise. In fact, they deliver the opposite: unhappiness and suffering. Instead of giving in to the desire, try moving back into awareness. Ask yourself,

Food Freedom And Truth

"Where is the quiet?" In this movement, you align with the intention that essence has for you—to experience the joy that comes from the quiet simplicity of this moment.

Desire: The Hydra

In Greek mythology, the hydra was a serpentlike water beast with many heads. When one of its heads was severed, two more would grow in its place. Desires are like the hydra's heads—when one desire is extinguished, another one immediately appears to take its place. But as human beings, we're programmed to miss the truth that striving to fulfill all of our desires is a pointless, unsatisfying, never-ending exercise. To keep us from seeing this truth, the ego encourages us to focus solely on the pleasure we believe will finally be ours when we get what we want.

A few years ago, I went on diet that was supposed to be the end of all diets. Spending a month on this highly restrictive diet was supposed to transform the body's metabolism such that it would stay naturally thin forever. At the end of the month, when my digital scale flashed back the number that had eluded me for 30 years, I was over the moon! I couldn't believe that I had finally done it. With a new, slinky body to flaunt, I was ecstatic…for the better part of five minutes.

Almost before I'd had a chance to register it, I got mentally caught up in doing whatever else the day held for me. Then it hit me: the realization that the joy of finally attaining what I thought I had wanted for so long, and the sense of accomplishment that it represented, were nowhere to be found. In their place were new problems, new desires to chase after (courtesy of the ego, of course). "If I could just solve these *new* problems," the ego assured me, "then I would finally have a happiness that would last."

Desires successfully motivate us to act because they promise lasting pleasure. In the moment we choose to follow a desire, we believe "If I can just get this one thing, I will be satisfied forever and not need to want again." But when we get what we want and summarily tick it off the list, we immediately move on to the next desire. Rather than providing us with endless pleasure, the minute we get what we thought we wanted, we forget about it or dismiss it, and a new thing becomes the sole focus of our attention.

As soon as you attain the body you have been coveting, the ego gives you another problem to fix. As soon as you get that first bit of chocolate cake into your mouth, the pleasure from it fades and you need to add another bite and then another to keep the pleasure going. You can't stop because the pleasure is so fleeting that if you do, it will end. The feeling of satisfaction slips through your fingers.

The ego functions just like the mythical hydra, only instead of generating new heads, the ego generates new desires. The moment we fulfill one desire, the ego makes sure another one grows up in its place. The truth about desire fulfillment is that there is no peace in it because whenever one of your dreams comes true, a new desire immediately arises to take its place.

The Truth about Desire

Exercise: Desire Fulfillment

Remember a time when you got something you really wanted. You won a prize, got the grade, finished a project, lost weight, won the boy's heart, or finally saved enough money to buy the house of your dreams. Remember what it felt like to be in the throes of the desire.

Now, think back on what it felt like to attain the desire.

Finally, what was it like five minutes or two days later? How long did the satisfaction of attaining the desire last? Did any new desires arise to take the place of the one you met?

Desire and Fear

Desire and fear work together to spawn the full range of emotions. As human beings, our most compelling desires are to survive and be loved. Desiring something that you don't have and that you believe you need in order to survive or be loved or that is necessary to your happiness, understandably creates fear. Fear leaves you angry, sad, guilty or ashamed, or all of those things. It can lead you to blame other people or feel resentful, envious or jealous.

The desire-fear combination can play out in very simple ways. Imagine perusing the menu at a restaurant and deciding on the vegetarian lasagna. Moments after you order, the waiter informs you that the kitchen is out of it. You feel disappointed because, when you made your selection, you created an image of it and imagined how good it would taste. That fantasy spawned a desire for the lasagna. Now, your expectation of the taste pleasure the lasagna will bring has been thwarted, and there's nothing you can do about it. For a moment, you're overcome with a feeling of disappointment and helplessness. This sounds like a small thing, but it's not.

Why does it matter so much? There's plenty of other tasty food in the kitchen. Yet somewhere, deep down, part of you believed that your happiness rested on getting that lasagna. Hearing that life had a different plan and lasagna wasn't part of it triggered a fear that now you won't be able to experience the pleasure you were hoping for. Your fantasy about the lasagna linked your happiness to the experience of tasting it. Not getting the lasagna is suddenly akin to being subjugated to a joyless existence for the rest of eternity.

The Truth about Desire

If we examined them, we would find that even the most petty desires, when they feel compelling, can be reduced to an underlying voice that says, "I'm afraid I'm not going to get what I need to survive, to be safe, loved or happy."

Now, imagine you're trying on a jacket. It fits you perfectly, and your mind travels to all the glorious events you'll attend wearing it. You decide to buy it. But as you slip it off, you notice that you misread the price tag. The number you see is way over your budget. You're flooded with disappointment, sadness and fear that you won't have anything to wear to those events if you don't buy the jacket—and that you won't be able to pay your bills if you do buy it.

This pain results from the subtle belief that you now need that jacket in order to feel safe, happy or okay, and your fear that you won't be able to get it. Before you saw the jacket, you didn't know you needed it. But now that you know it exists, you've created a desire that is causing you to suffer.

Next, use your imagination to take the fear of not getting the jacket to the worst possible outcome. If you don't get the jacket, you won't be admired. In addition, the people you want to impress at the functions you'd wear the jacket to will reject you. Then what? If you don't make a good impression, you won't get the job opportunity you were hoping for. Then what? Without a new, higher-paying job, you won't be able to buy a house and without a house, you're a failure. Everyone knows that owning a house means that you've arrived and are successful. And there you have it. In your mind, the difference between having that jacket and not having it is the difference between success and failure in life. And if you're a failure, you might as well be dead. No wonder the idea of not getting the jacket triggers powerful emotions—at the root of it is the fear of death.

Now take all of those thoughts and conclusions to inquiry by asking yourself if they are true. Is it really true that you won't have anything to wear to the functions if you don't buy the jacket? Is it really true that people will reject you or fail to admire you if you're not wearing that particular jacket? Is it really true that you'll be a failure if you don't own a house?

This inquiry can help you see that even if all your fears come to pass, you'll still be okay. You can still be happy. This realization releases the air from the pumped-up emotional balloon of desire and fear. We are only at their effect when we don't question them, and christen them with belief instead.

Beliefs give rise to emotions that feel powerful and real because they manifest as sensations in the body very quickly. Before we can ask, "What in the world just happened?" we're elbow deep in last night's lemon chiffon pie. But even when that happens, there's no harm done. Even when you've reached for food or overeaten pleasure food because of the desire-fear duo, it's never too late to dissect and inquire into what just happened. The more you do this, the more conscious you will become and, eventually, you won't create the desires and fears. If you do, you'll see through them so quickly that you'll easily be able to interrupt your emotional eating reaction.

Caught Between Two Opposing Egoic Desires

When we romanticize food and thin bodies, we're caught between two opposing egoic desires: wanting to experience the taste pleasure of rich, decadent food and wanting to be admired for having a slim body. It's challenging enough to have one desire, but to have two powerful desires that are inherently contradictory is a huge challenge. We drive ourselves insane by dieting to get the ideal body and, at the same time, convince ourselves that we're deprived because we can't eat the pleasure food we crave, all while the ego delights in how busy she's keeping us. Once we believe the deprivation thought, it's not long before we rebel and frantically race to the nearest donut shop.

We want a thin body not because being slimmer means we'll feel better, be healthier, or live longer, but because our culture tells us that thinner bodies are more attractive to others. The prospect of being admired drives the ego to strive tirelessly to reach its goal of a sexy body. According to the ego, possessing a beautiful body delivers a successful material life. The ego reveres surface values and appearances like wealth, power, youth and physical beauty. Intangibles such as the spiritual qualities that essence embodies—compassion, kindness and patience—don't rate because you can't see them or touch them.

The ego tells us that when we attain the body of our dreams, not only will we revel in our reflection in the full-length mirror and look forward to shopping for bathing suits, but also finally snare the perfect life and relationship. The ego hypothesizes that the appearance of a perfect outward life means everlasting happiness on the inside, just like in fairytales.

The only problem with striving to attain a thin body is that it precludes eating the pleasure foods we crave. We can abide this imagined deprivation for a short time—enough time to lose the fat covering the slinky body of our dreams—but when the excess pounds melt away, all bets are off. It's celebration time. That's when the pleasure-seeking child coaxes us with rationalizations like "You deserve some pleasure after losing all that weight. You've been so good. If you gain a little back, so what? You can just diet it off tomorrow."

Why is it that the first thing we want to do when we've lost our excess weight is celebrate with the food we've had to give up in order to lose the weight? If we have a habit of romanticizing food, we associate it with pleasure and celebration. If food has been our main source of pleasure, it's natural for us to return to it after we've lost weight. If we want to stop doing that, however, we have to fundamentally change our relationship with food by changing the way we think about it. Simply starting a new exercise routine or going on a diet doesn't solve the core issue, which is the misguided way we think about food.

To be free, we have to see the whole truth about these two egoic desires: neither can bring lasting happiness. The whole truth about pleasure food is that its nice taste is fleeting and the negative consequences of overeating it can last for hours, days or weeks. The whole truth about the body of your dreams is that even if you attain it, not all of your problems will be solved. It might even create some new problems. For example, attracting more attention may have its downsides. People who are interested in you because you look a certain way may not be capable of the deep connection your heart longs for. And attracting more attention may force you to confront intimacy issues that you had been avoiding.

In addition, the truth about bodies is that, no matter how beautiful they are, they age. They get old and sick, and eventually die. Why would you devote considerable time, energy and money to a futile pursuit like trying to hold onto a particular appearance when bodies have such a destiny? Why not spend your energy and time on that which is supremely pleasurable and can never be taken from you—your very own true self? It's timeless, ageless, indestructible and always available to you. When you put your attention on essence, eventually you come to rest there and identify as it, rather than as a body. In this way, you become invulnerable to life's variability. Problems can't touch you and desires don't even bother to arise. You come to know yourself as supreme freedom, and abide in your own heart, living out the rest of your days in this world but not of it.

Desire, Cravings and the Future

The most common question I'm asked in my work is "Can you help me deal with my cravings?" People tell me they can eat moderately for a while, but then a monster craving hits and their resolve turns to goo. "I'm helpless," they say, because when a craving strikes, they imagine that they have to seek out and consume whatever food they're craving *right then*.

To begin to disempower food cravings, take a look at how they operate. Your desire for taste pleasure and the fear of missing out on it arise simultaneously. This tag team of desire and fear keeps you bouncing back and forth in a fantasy that was created by the ego. You imagine the moment of pleasure that you assume will result once you obtain the object of your desire, which triggers a fear that you'll miss out on that pleasure if you don't obtain it.

The ego stirs up cravings to try to convince you to go after what you want right now in order to keep you out of the present moment, where cravings *don't exist*. This is counterintuitive. But when you're focused on a promise of pleasure that's right around the corner, you're in the realm of imagination, not in the present. The ego knows that if you delay acting on a craving for even a moment, it risks losing your attention. That moment is an opportunity for you to become distracted by reality and move out of the mind and into essence. For the ego, your moving into essence is a plight worse than death, because in essence, the ego doesn't exist.

You may think you're addicted to food, but the truth is, you're addicted to your fantasies about food. These fantasies about taste pleasure are so seductive because they allow you to transcend the principle of duality that links pleasure with pain.

The Truth about Desire

Transported by the mind, you enter a world where you can opt for only the pleasurable aspect of an experience and leave out the pain. Your fantasies never tell the whole truth about getting what you want. They allow you to pick the part of your experience that you want and omit the rest. If your fantasies told the whole truth about experience and included both pleasure and pain, they couldn't hook you in the same way.

The other reason a craving can have so much power is that a fantasy of a future moment can be very captivating, particularly if the present moment isn't delivering the kind of experience you had been hoping for. The cost is that you miss out on the aliveness that comes from experiencing what is here right now without the filter of the mind. Because you can pay attention to only one thing at a time, thinking about the future blocks your ability to experience the present moment and allows the ego to maintain its position of control. As enticing as it is to imagine a future reality that contains all of what you want and nothing that you don't want, ultimately, the world of the imagination is flat and unsatisfying, like watching the same movie over and over again. If you know everything that is going to happen, you're robbed of life's freshness and fun.

When you are present, and step back into essence, an irrepressible joy and feeling of "all is well" envelops you. Perhaps it doesn't get your pulse racing like cravings do, but it is fulfilling and juicy in a way that a fantasy can never be. Being aligned with essence not only has no downside, it actually rescues you from experiencing the downside of following a craving. When you are in the throes of a craving, remind yourself of this truth: cravings come from the ego in child mode. The child hooks you with a sliver of truth about

Food Freedom And Truth

pleasure food—that it tastes good—but leaves out all of the negative consequences.

When a craving strikes, take a moment and move your attention back to essence by reminding yourself that you are that which is aware of the desire for food. You can never be the desire. Step back into alignment with your true identity and move your attention out of the ego's reach, where you are no longer vulnerable to it. Shift out of your mind-generated fantasy and into the present moment, the bastion of joy and peace. Realize that, contrary to the ego's promise of happiness through desire fulfillment, this is the only place that truly satisfies the purpose of human life.

Exercise: Moving into the Present Moment

Take some deep breaths and become acutely attentive to what is arising in your awareness in this moment. What sounds, smells, sights or body sensations do you notice? This moment contains a whole host of experiences if you are present enough to notice them. However, if you're caught up in fantasies about a possible future moment, you miss what is here right now. You miss your life and opt for an imaginary existence.

To shift out of your mind, reenter reality through your senses by noticing what you are aware of in this moment. Do this periodically during your day today when you notice that you're caught up in thought.

How to Stop Creating Negative Emotions and Cravings

To see how it's possible to stop creating negative emotions and cravings, imagine that you're going through your day and notice a stressful thought arising—life is hard. Because you're engaged in a household chore that you find boring, you decide that the thought is true. Believing the thought breathes life into it and generates unhappy feelings. Instantly, you dismiss all the times when life has been effortless and joyful. You assume that the sliver of truth in the stressful thought, that life can feel challenging and unpleasant sometimes, describes the totality of your life experience—and you run to the pantry for something sweet to change your present experience. You completely forget how sweet and gratifying it feels to face challenges and grow.

As soon as you buy into that negative belief about life, you identify and merge with it, creating a negative emotion. That emotion can cause you to feel powerless, hopeless or angry at life. If you eat emotionally, oftentimes a negative emotion creates a craving, a frantic, powerful desire to find and consume pleasure food.

Stymieing this mechanism of negative emotion and craving creation requires you to become aware of your thoughts. Most thoughts are neutral, arising and subsiding virtually unnoticed. But because of your specific life experiences and the conclusions you've come to as a result of them, some negative thoughts catch your attention and hook you right away. That's because they reinforce your negative conditioning—the negative beliefs you already have about yourself.

Throughout the years, you have strengthened these beliefs by believing them every time they arise, thereby generating painful emotions. Because life's plan is to keep triggering that conditioning until you heal it, you can support life's intention for you in two ways: by practicing inquiry and by catching these thoughts before they turn into emotions.

When you are in a situation that usually triggers you, pay special attention to the stressful thoughts that arise. By realizing that any stressful thought is actually a lie, you have an opportunity to interrupt your usual pattern of generating negative feelings. You simply notice a stressful thought and stop yourself from christening it with belief. You notice it, instantly realize that it's not true, and turn away from it. The next time a stressful thought bubbles up, try saying to yourself, "This thought is a lie because it doesn't tell the whole truth." That frees you of it. No belief is formed and no emotion is created.

The Stickiness of a Food Desire

If you're like me and food has been the love of your life, a food desire can seem overwhelming and virtually impossible to ignore. We're programmed to listen to and follow our desires, and if you have a belief that food is your greatest source of pleasure and happiness, then food desires are particularly powerful.

When a craving, which is really the thought "I want," arises, it generates desire. Along with the desire comes urgency, the belief that following this desire is a life-or-death imperative that can't wait. A food desire can feel so powerful that you're convinced you must follow it right now; otherwise, you'll be miserable, stuck in a craving hell for all eternity.

Food Freedom And Truth

The pleasure-seeking child creates these desires based on the assumption that obtaining the object of your desire will lead to happiness. She pretends to be very wise, coaxing you to live life her way and follow her desires. If you do this, she promises, you'll be happy and your life will turn out the way you've always wanted it to.

The Buddha suggests something very different: that all desires bring suffering. If you follow a desire, even though it promises happiness, what you find on the other end of the desire is not what you expect. Either you get what you want, then immediately take it for granted while another desire springs up in its place or you get what you want, but the pleasure you get from it also leads to pain.

The child, of course, insists that she's only trying to help you feel better. Life feels frustrating, stressful or overwhelming, or your friend said something unkind about you to another friend, or you forget a file you need and have to run back to work unexpectedly. At those moments, the child rides in on a white horse, offering a well-deserved respite from life's little or not-so-little annoyances. "What's so wrong with trying to distract yourself from an uncomfortable feeling through food?" she asks.

There's nothing wrong with having a little party with food (emphasis on "little") every once in a while. But if that's how you habitually relate to food, as a source of comfort and entertainment, you will eventually pay the price: ill health, low self-esteem and a heavier body.

The bottom line is that when we go after desires, it's like stepping in chewing gum. Desires come with gooey strings attached that stick with us as we walk down the street of life.

The Truth about Desire

Their negative effects stay with us much longer than the fleeting pleasure they offer.

The ego lies to us about following our desires, and about our food desires, in particular. Following them does not bring happiness; it actually creates unhappiness. Yet we're programmed to follow them. Eventually, we evolve out of this pattern by seeing the whole truth: that desire never delivers on its promise.

Thankfully, when we're ready, we discover that happiness is our nature. It's always available for us to notice, revel in and live from. When we listen to the ego's "if-thens," we suffer: "If only I could have that taste in my mouth, then I would be happy. If only I could eat as much of my favorite foods as I wanted and not get fat, then I would be happy." The if-then equation doesn't work for happiness because happiness is always right here, right now. The statement "If I get X, then I will be happy" takes you into the future. Because life only happens now, there is no life in the future. It stands to reason that happiness can't live there either.

The nature of happiness is quite different from what the ego leads us to believe. It's not a prize. It's not something that is manufactured or achieved. Rather, it's omnipresent, available in any moment when you move out of thought or feeling and give the present moment your attention. It's so simple! And this simple way of living leaves the ego without a job. So, the next time the child tempts you with a food desire, remember the whole truth about the nature of desire. It's all trumped up and doesn't deliver. Yes, following a desire will provide a few fleeting moments of taste pleasure, but it's always followed by hours and possibly days of misery.

Mastering Desire

Perhaps you're reading this book because, like most people, you've been living at the effect of your desires and believe that you have no choice but to follow them when they arise. In other words, your desires have been mastering you. Maybe you believe that your eating, weight and body-image issues are your curse, a cruel joke of the creator. Yet hidden within these issues is a wonderful gift: the possibility of not just evolving out of the suffering food, eating and weight have caused you, but of waking up out of ego-generated suffering altogether. Healing could mean living out the rest of your days in the heavenly state called "happy for no reason."

There comes a time in everyone's evolution when playing the ego's game just doesn't cut it anymore. That time came for me after 35 years of feasting and fasting, shame, blame and self-deprecation. My hope is that you will be smarter than I was, and embrace the tools of self-inquiry and meditation that lead you to greater joy and freedom, and to the truth of your being. As you begin using these tools, you'll stop being cannon fodder for the ego.

The first step to mastering desire is realizing when you're identified with your thoughts. The realization brings you into witness mode. The second step is turning away from those thoughts and doing or thinking about something else or simply hanging out in the thought-free state by focusing on what you are hearing, seeing or smelling. In Zen, this process is called "the backwards step." It means moving out of ordinary consciousness, where you're identified with the thoughts and feelings that arise, and stepping back into witness consciousness, where you're aligned with that which is aware

The Truth about Desire

of the thoughts and feelings. When a desire arises, you simply label it as a thought, and say to yourself, "It's just a thought. It's not me. How could it be me? I'm over here noticing it."

It's really like doing anything else that you've done that's challenging. It's like when you were a kid and the other kids in the neighborhood asked you to come out and play, but you had homework to do. Turning away from a desire is like deciding to do your homework. You put play out of your mind and focus on your homework. Otherwise, you'll suffer and not be able to do either.

Overcoming desire is not about fighting your ego. That's a battle you can never win. It's about engaging the adult, rational part of yourself that doesn't want to cause you needless suffering. Fortunately for us, the ego has never had any power, thoughts have never had any power and desire has never had any power. You just innocently got lost in the illusion and forgot that you, not your ego, have always had all the power. Along with most of the human race, you loaned your power to your thoughts and desires and then believed that you were powerless in their presence and had no choice but to follow them.

Now that you know how things work, you can choose where to put your attention and what to believe. You have the power to turn your attention away from a desire. And when you do that, you see that it's merely a phantom, not the omnipotent force of nature you took it for. At first, turning away from your desires may be easier said than done, particularly if you have, over the years, reinforced the habit of following them. But since you have all the power, all the time, you can form a new habit of following the truth instead.

Exercise: Mastering Desire

Start by taking an internal stand to both let go of your old habit of following desires and form a new habit of consciously choosing to do what makes sense from the wise, mature part of yourself.

Next, practice by using a dress rehearsal. A dress rehearsal is imagining that an impractical food desire is on the scene. See yourself recognizing it by saying, "Oh that's just the child. For a moment there, I thought I was the child. I thought I wanted what she wanted." You can use a memory of your last emotional eating attack to help you do this exercise. Simply imagine yourself consciously dis-identifying with the thought "I want" and stepping back into awareness.

Then, see yourself focusing on whatever else was arising in that moment other than the "I want" thought. What were you seeing, hearing, smelling? What were the sensations in that moment? Reengage in what you were doing.

The Truth about Desire

It took me an entire year to be able to turn away from a desire to eat emotionally. So don't worry if it takes a long time for you to be conscious enough to turn away from a desire for food. In the meantime, if you do follow a food desire and find yourself eating emotionally, remember to go easy on yourself about it. It's natural. Resist any impulse to beat yourself up about it. Simply use it as an opportunity to practice a dress rehearsal.

Consciousness will start coming in earlier and earlier when the "I want" thought arises. At first, it will come in after your emotional eating attack, then toward the end, then in the middle and then in the beginning. Pretty soon, you'll find yourself looking down as your hand reaches for food and saying to yourself, "Wait a minute. The child is on the scene. It's not me. I really don't want to follow this desire right now because I'll feel bad if I do."

After a bit more time, you might notice your feet climbing the stairs toward the kitchen for no good reason, and then find yourself directing them to climb back down. You might notice some emotional weather moving across the sky of your being, followed by an image of an apple fritter, and then say to yourself, "Oops, there's a food fantasy," and instantly turn away from it. In time, you'll be able to stop chasing after these desires and living at their effect as you assume your rightful position of power and mastery.

THE TRUTH ABOUT BELIEFS

The sense "I am" is always with you, only you have attached all kinds of things to it—body, feelings, thoughts, ideas, possessions, etc. All these self-identifications are misleading. Because of them, you take yourself to be what you are not.
   —Nisargadatta Maharaj

The Birth of a Core Belief

In childhood, when something upsetting happens, it's often our natural response to form a negative, painful conclusion called a core belief. A client of mine we'll call Sarah once shared that she often felt invisible growing up. She said that as a child, she would frequently sit at the dinner table in silence while the rest of her family engaged in lively conversation. She related a story about a particular day when her family and her mother's boyfriend, "Sam," were all sitting together in the living room. When Sarah didn't understand a rather sophisticated joke Sam made, Sam called her stupid and her entire family, including her mother, laughed. From that day forward, every time he saw her, Sam would call out, "Hey, stupid!"

Like most children, Sarah was very willing to believe what adults told her, and she concluded that she was, in fact, stupid. After all, the people closest to her, who were supposed to love her the most, had laughed at her, not with her. If they considered her to be an object of ridicule, certainly the rest of the world would agree. That was how her core belief was formed.

Because of this belief, she felt inferior to other people and, as she grew older, carefully avoided situations that would draw attention to her. Sarah's core belief was now stored as conditioning, a "button" just waiting to be pushed at some future time. The experience of her whole family, including her mother, laughing at her, coupled with Sam's continual reinforcement of the belief every time he saw her, hurt so much that, without realizing it, Sarah spent years trying to protect herself from ever having to experience the pain associated with it. The last thing she wanted was to experience that hurt and humiliation again.

Because all attention had the potential to become negative attention, at school, Sarah avoided the spotlight. Whereas some children with the core belief "I'm stupid" might avoid academics and devote themselves to playing sports—figuring that no one will expect an athlete to be smart—Sarah tried to become an academic overachiever. She did her homework twice, so she would get only positive feedback from her teachers. But, try as she might, she could not commandeer life away from any triggers of her core belief.

Sarah told me that, throughout her adulthood, she had always assumed she had to work harder than everyone else did in order to stay employed. In spite of this, she found jobs where her bosses ridiculed her and did not respect her talents or intelligence. She worked until 9:00 p.m. every evening, when her coworkers with the same salary left at 5:00 p.m. It didn't occur to her to protest or ask for help because she believed that she needed to work harder to make up for her inferiority. She assumed that her bosses and coworkers believed what she believed about herself.

The truth was that Sarah's bosses were just providing "triggering services," pushing that button that existed inside of her. Secretly, she believed that they were right, which is why she didn't challenge them or look for another job. "All bosses are slave drivers and every company exploits their employees like this one," she convinced herself. This is how many of us react in button-pushing situations. Conditioned by the ego to march into battle the instant we're triggered, we get caught up in stories that reinforce the core beliefs we formed in childhood, causing ourselves even more suffering.

The Truth about Emotions

Uncovering Core Beliefs

It's helpful to uncover negative core beliefs we formed in childhood in order to ascertain whether they're true. Only by seeing them for the lies they are can we ultimately become free of them. Asking whether our core beliefs are true is one form of inquiry, but we need to identify what those beliefs are before we can examine them. To discover them, we have to become truth sleuths, and take a close look at any errant painful beliefs that may have left their footprints on our consciousness.

The first clue that a painful belief is operating is any emotional discomfort in our system. When a core belief is triggered, it hurts so much because it reinforces the original childhood trauma that first created it, and our body tells us we've been triggered through its immediate contraction. Out of the blue, we can be suddenly overcome with intense sadness, fear, anger, frustration, resentment or depression, all of which can indicate that we believed a negative thought, identified with it, and unconsciously allowed it to take root in our body.

Once we've formed a core belief that there is something terribly wrong with us, we try to protect ourselves from ever having to experience the pain associated with it. We do this by (consciously or unconsciously) trying to avoid situations that we think might trigger it. Yet despite our most valiant efforts to sidestep situations that trigger us, life experiences eventually bring us face to face with them. When someone criticizes us using words that remotely resemble a core belief, we are overcome with unbearable feelings.

Interestingly, core beliefs explain why certain comments trigger one person, but have no impact on someone else. If you have the core belief "I'm stupid," when someone says, "Wow, you were really slow on the uptake," you probably get very upset. However, if you believe you are intelligent, the same remark might not even register. You might view it as curious but not worth your attention. Or you might acknowledge that you were, in fact, slow on the uptake in a given moment, without taking it personally.

Eleanor Roosevelt's famous saying "No one can make you feel inferior without your consent" is a profound commentary on core beliefs and the situations that trigger them—because no one can push a button that we didn't first create and plant in our own psyche. When someone pushes our buttons, it's as if they're saying, "Yes, I agree with you. The core belief you formed about yourself in early childhood is correct." And they don't even have to get the wording right. Even if what they're saying doesn't match our core belief, if they come close, we assume that they agree with it. If there is any contrary information, we filter it out, like propaganda machines choosing only the statistics that support our core belief and ignoring the rest.

If you have the core belief that you can't do anything right, a minor constructive suggestion from a friend, even if it's delicately handled, can set you off. If you're convinced that you're overweight and don't look good in clothes, and your partner doesn't compliment you on a new outfit, it pushes your "I'm too fat button." You see the failure to notice your new outfit as tacit agreement with the belief. Your partner's behavior may have nothing to do with agreeing or disagreeing with your body image. Perhaps he's worried about losing a big account at work or has a splitting headache. When it comes to button pushing, we need other people to supply only a few lines. Then, we fill in the rest of the story.

The Truth about Emotions

This is because the fear of annihilation is embedded in every core belief. We have a fear of losing who we think we are. To our psyche, it's literally a matter of life and death when our buttons are pushed, which is why we react so violently. We would rather die than experience the feelings it triggers in us. Accordingly, we may use food to escape or to distract or comfort ourselves, repeating a habit most likely begun in childhood. A dreaded core belief about ourselves surfaces and, if it has been our pattern to eat emotionally, we reach for food.

Although we can't rewrite history or erase painful events from our memories, we can rewrite the conclusions we came to about these events. The next time you suspect a core belief has been triggered, try simply asking yourself, "What did I just tell myself that caused me to feel bad?" Your answer can help uncover a core belief you formed in childhood that is negatively influencing your life to this day.

To create a healing environment for the core belief, try staying present with, rather than acting on, the emotions and sensations that have flooded you, while inquiring into the beliefs that triggered them. If you can do this without any agenda to have the feeling dissipate, insights will often arise to help you heal the belief and free yourself from the conditioning that triggered you. Being with the feeling is like saying "I want the truth," and this attitude invites insights and understanding.

We can debunk our core beliefs through the inquiry process (outlined on page XX) and eventually render them powerless. In this way, we can avoid creating the emotions that continually cause us to run to the refrigerator. Liberating ourselves from the debilitating emotions triggered by core beliefs frees us to engage freshly and cleanly in each moment, and to connect with the aliveness and joy that is our birthright.

Exercise: Uncovering Your Core Beliefs

Scan your childhood and your current life for painful experiences that might have led you to create core beliefs. What conclusions did you come to as a result of these experiences? Using a stream of consciousness approach, record these conclusions, taking note of the ones that possess the greatest emotional charge. These are your core beliefs.

Then, ask yourself how they have impacted you throughout your life. What decisions have you made based on these beliefs? What actions have you taken or not taken as a result of these beliefs?

You Are More Powerful than Your Conditioning

When a negative emotion erupts in your awareness, because it manifests as a strong sensation in your body, it can leave you feeling powerless and small. In order for you to experience the emotion, you must have inadvertently believed the painful thought that generated it. Hence, you are at the mercy of both the painful belief and the emotion, and, if it has been your habit, you'll likely look to food to give you some relief.

In spite of how it feels, you are much more powerful than any of your conditioning. As a spiritual being with human conditioning, there's always the potential for this conditioning to be triggered and to create unhappiness, particularly if you buy into the belief that your life is fraught with problems. However, if you interrupt the programming that caused you to believe your negative thoughts and merge with the feelings they generate, you can create an entirely different experience and relationship with life—an entirely different life.

When you are identified with your ego, you feel vulnerable and separate, and you resist life. Finding that you are not able to control life and bend it to your will, you create problems for yourself over and over again. Yet, from the larger perspective of living in this world as a spiritual being that enjoys and learns from all experiences, so many of the things that you considered to be problems in the past are no longer issues for you. When you trust that the same power that turns acorns into mighty oak trees is operating through you, you can relax, and let life move you, rather than trying to make life happen through your will. It's all a matter of perspective.

Food, Freedom, and Truth

When you find yourself in an untenable situation, you can notice whether you feel moved to take action to change it or not. If you don't feel moved to change it from the outside, rather than telling yourself an unhappy story about it as you might have in the past, you can approach it with openness and curiosity to see what new learning life has brought you. You don't have to like the situation that is appearing, but it's irrational not to accept it. Because the situation is here right now and nothing can change that fact.

As a spiritual being, the people you believed to be the bane of your existence aren't a problem for you anymore because you stop taking their behavior personally. If there's something in your relationship with a certain person that points you back to your own conditioning, see it as a gift. Look at the underlying belief that's causing your suffering, and liberate it through inquiry.

As for anything else in a particular interaction, take responsibility for your part in it and let the rest of it go. Realize that when people appear to be having a problem with you, they're most likely just reacting to their own conditioning. This, of course, has nothing to do with you. In the past, you might have fed your reactions to people and situations with food, but now you needn't have any reaction. You don't have to soothe yourself because you haven't wounded yourself by believing untrue, painful thoughts.

As a spiritual being, you're more powerful than your conditioning—because you created it. And as its creator, you have the power to debunk it and see through it, not just once or twice, but over and over and over again. Eventually, through your vigilance and your willingness to stop following your painful thinking, your conditioning will dissolve and, with it, any power to create negative emotions.

Negative Self-Talk

Recently, a friend of mine talked to me about how he wanted to manage his eating. He began by saying, "You know, I've always been a little bit lazy." The words rolled so trippingly off his tongue that they caught me off guard and I fell under their spell. For a split second, I actually believed him. In fact, when I thought more about it, I recalled that he'd frequently said things like that in the past, if not in the same words, then variations on that theme.

Ego talk is like riveting propaganda. It's mesmerizing. Afterward you hear it, to come back to yourself, you may need to metaphorically splash your face with cold water to shake off its effects. If you tell people the same thing repeatedly, eventually, you wear them down and they believe you. Political machines know this ego trick well. In fascist regimes throughout history, we've witnessed the effectiveness of repetition in getting whole populations to believe propaganda. Another trick is telling people something true, hooking them with that truth, winning their trust or buy-in, and then piling on partial truths and the lies. That often works, too.

We may not be ruled by a totalitarian regime, but inside our heads, we have our very own ranting fascist dictator, who uses the same highly effective tactics that the bad guys have used for centuries. When we tell ourselves that we're lazy or lack self-control or anything else that's negative, we're acting as the ego's mouthpiece. We rattle off negative self-talk as if it's actually true.

Our core beliefs are stories that we've been writing about ourselves since childhood. As a result of years of repetition and reinforcement, we've come to believe these core beliefs are accurate representations of who we are. Because we now accept them, we no longer question them, in the same way the German people, once under the spell of the Nazi party line, no longer questioned its motives or message or agenda. The ego's self-talk is no less insidious or destructive.

Here's a quick rule of thumb: If you're telling yourself something negative and it makes you feel bad, you can know that it comes from the ego and is not true. Just because you have a history of telling yourself this story and believing it doesn't make it any less a lie.

Here are the questions I pose to my friend: "You're a little lazy—is that true? Can you absolutely know it's true? Could the opposite statement, that you're not lazy, be as true or more true? What's your evidence for that? What are the examples?" I know my friend. If he answers these questions truthfully, "lazy" is the last descriptor he'll pin to himself.

If, during your life, you have regularly engaged in negative self-talk, it may take some doing to break the habit. The cost of not breaking it, however, is steep: allowing it to continue to ravage your self-esteem. Living with chronic low self-esteem means that you have limited your choices and avoided risks that could have brought you much pleasure and growth.

Although it may not sound spiritually correct, to counteract this tendency, I recommend that you fake it till you make it. Act as if you are precious and valuable to the unfolding of consciousness. This is the truth. Life needs you to make your unique contribution to the whole. And if you don't do it, no one else can.

In addition, make a point of asking for help to be able to notice your negative self-talk. This is not as easy as it sounds,

Food, Freedom, and Truth

particularly if you've never tried to become aware of or question your negative self-talk. You may be surprised at how often you say harsh things to yourself.

Next, when you say something critical to yourself, turn this comment around to its opposite, and support the opposite statement with at least three concrete examples. This practice debunks the original negative statement, weakens it and, eventually, if you're vigilant, squashes it once and for all. Even when you miss opportunities to interrupt your negative self-talk, be gentle with yourself about it. You're interrupting a long-standing, deeply entrenched pattern that may take some time to heal.

Complexes

Painful beliefs don't exist in isolation. Whenever you find one, you're likely to discover many others that are related. These interrelated beliefs are emotional complexes that form our negative self-images. Uncovering core beliefs and mapping complexes is the first step in realizing the freedom that is your birthright. It's the first step in releasing the suffering created by your conditioning and the feelings attached to it. Some examples of commonly held core beliefs are: I'm no good, life is unfair, I'm a failure, nothing ever works out for me, no one cares about me, no one will ever love me, I'll never get it right, I can't stick with things.

Think about one of your own core beliefs. When you're feeling down on yourself, what tapes run through your head? What do you say to yourself that makes you feel bad? When you find a core belief that resonates for you, map out the complex by sitting with paper and pen in hand and allowing yourself to relax and breathe deeply. From this relaxed place, allow your mind to wander. As beliefs arise in your consciousness, log them.

Use the diagram on the next page to help you map out the complex you're uncovering. On a sheet of paper, place the negative core belief in the middle of the page. Then, draw lines radiating off that belief for any ancillary beliefs that seem to be related.

After you find one belief, keep looking. You're probably not going to uncover the whole complex or heal the feelings attached to each belief in one sitting. But the next time that feeling or belief comes up, investigate it, and see what other beliefs are attached to it. You might discover entirely new beliefs that you didn't see before.

One of my particularly potent beliefs used to be "I'm a screw-up." I wrote that in the middle of my page and created lines extending from it. Some of the other beliefs that arose from it were: "I'm not important," "I'm boring," "No one that I find interesting will be interested in me," "I'll be rejected when someone more interesting comes along," "I'm worthless" and "I'm invisible." To disable this complex of mine, I used inquiry to question each belief in the complex.

To weaken your own complex, simply identify the beliefs and sub-beliefs so that you can begin to dissolve it using inquiry. Healing a complex takes vigilance, investigating and inquiring over and over again. Eventually, as you pick it apart, it will weaken and dissolve.

Exercise: Mapping a Complex

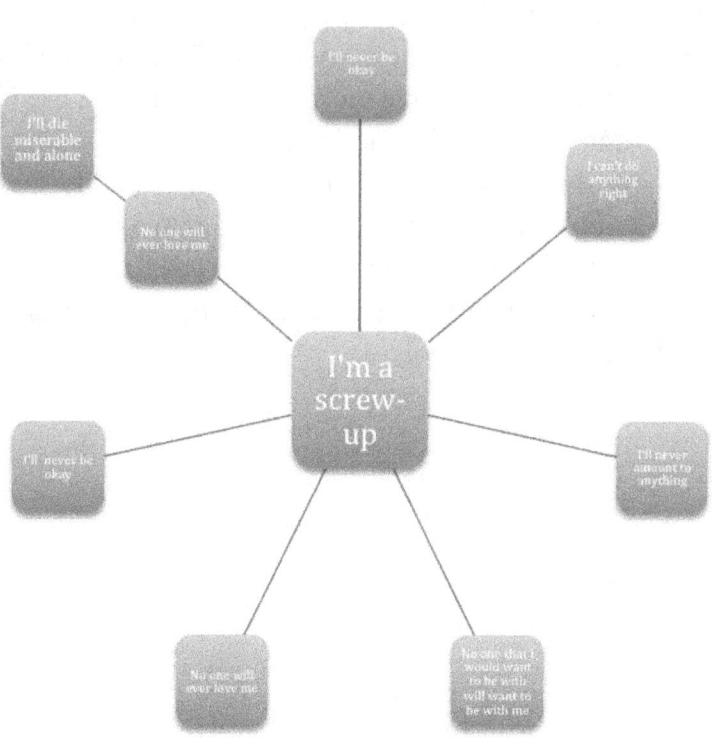

Kryptonite for Core Beliefs

It's possible that, without realizing it, you've been navigating your life and relationships to avoid triggering your core beliefs. Life, however, doesn't allow that. There is no hiding. Whether you like it or not, life puts you in situations that trigger your core beliefs so that you can heal and evolve. To free yourself from living at the effect of core beliefs, support your evolutionary impulse to heal and stop eating emotionally, you have to see that your core beliefs aren't true.

There is great power in using inquiry to see the falseness of a belief. In many cases, this seeing is enough to undo conditioning. The inquiry I recommend, now that you have used the mapping technique outlined in the last section to uncover you core beliefs and their sub-beliefs is from *The Work* by Byron Katie, and it's comprised of four questions and a turnaround.

The first step is to pick a stressful belief to work on. Here is example of how you would use *The Work* to debunk the belief, "I am unlovable."

Belief: I am unlovable.

Next ask yourself the these four questions about the belief:

1. Is it true? *Yes*
2. Can you absolutely know that it's true? *No*
3. How do you react, what happens, when you believe that thought? *I feel sad and hopeless. I believe that I'm doomed to an unhappy, loveless existence. I don't take care of myself because I don't think I'm worth it. I think negative thoughts about myself. I isolate and avoid social situations. I withhold my*

love because I'm afraid that no one will receive it or return it. I eat too much.

4. Who would you be without that thought? *I would be someone who loves myself and loves life. Because I love myself, it would be natural for me to express my love to others and think only kind thoughts about myself. Because I value myself, it would be natural for me to take care of myself by resting, taking time to feed my soul and eating healthily. Without that thought, I would be comfortable in my own skin, free and happy.*

Turn around the belief you are questioning (to yourself and to the opposite of your thinking) and be sure to find at least three genuine examples of each turnaround. You won't necessarily be able to use all three turnarounds for each belief.

To the opposite: I am lovable.
    1. My daughter loves me.
    2. My dog loves me.
    3. My father and sisters love me.
    4. My girlfriends love me.
To my thinking: My thinking is unlovable.
    1. The thought "I am unlovable" is not loving.
    2. Often my thoughts about myself are critical and, therefore, not loving.
    3. Often my thoughts are negative in general and, therefore, not loving. I can see that my thinking is unlovable because when I have this negative mindset, it makes it hard for me to be happy and enjoy life.

Food, Freedom, and Truth

Now it's your turn. List one of the beliefs you uncovered on a sheet of paper. Be sure to choose one that has a great deal of emotional charge for you. Then, ask yourself these four questions about it:

1. Is it true?
2. Can you absolutely know that it's true?
3. How do you react, what happens, when you believe that thought?
4. Who would you be without that thought?

Turn around the concept you are questioning (to yourself, to the opposite or to your thinking) and be sure to find at least three genuine examples of each turnaround.

The Truth about Emotions

Exercise: Inquiry

Get out your notebook and chose a particularly charged belief from your map to use for your inquiry. Write the belief across the top of your page and record your answers to the four questions and the turnaround.

Here are the four questions and the turnaround from The Work:

1. Is it true?
2. Can you absolutely know that it's true?
3. How do you react, what happens, when you believe that thought?
4. Who would you be without that thought?

Turn around the concept you are questioning (to yourself and to the opposite of your thinking) and be sure to find at least three genuine examples of each turnaround.

The impact of this simple inquiry is atomic. It enables you to experience the truth that no painful belief is true. Answering these questions is a way to prove to yourself that the beliefs that have been guiding your eating and many other areas of your life have no credence. Inquiry allows you to lift the veil of self-delusion and expose the ego for what it is: a compulsive liar.

It's possible that simply seeing an untruth will be enough to cause the conditioning to drop away. Indeed, inquiry is powerful because it can bring immediate results without much practice or skill. Odd as it may sound, it uses the mind to go beyond the mind. It uses the rational mind to see through the fallacies that the egoic mind perpetrates. We don't mean to lie

The Truth about Emotions

to ourselves, it's just that we've been programmed to and so it takes some alertness on our part to say, "Wait a minute. Just because this thought just flashed across my mind doesn't mean it's true."

For many people, seeing a deeply entrenched belief as a lie just once probably won't be enough to heal it. When you have an issue that you've struggled with repeatedly, disempowering it means repeatedly unraveling, investigating and releasing it. True freedom requires vigilance, the willingness to witness a lie over and over again. Each time a core belief arises, rather than following it and feeding it with more thoughts, simply notice it, and see the untruth of it. Then, reinforce this seeing with all the reasons why the belief is untrue. Over time, this repetition permanently disables belief. The failsafe method for rendering core beliefs powerless is to repeatedly use inquiry to *stop believing in them.* Inquiry is kryptonite for core beliefs.

When you feel anything other than happy, relaxed and at peace, you can know that you believed a painful thought. When you discover the painful story or belief that you bought into that caused you to feel bad, take it to inquiry so it can release its grip on you, allowing you to once again rest in the joy of your true nature.

The Relationship Between Inquiry and Food Issues

What does inquiry have to do with becoming free of food, eating and weight issues? Everything. Using food to comfort and entertain yourself means that your thinking about it must be inaccurate and deluded. I say this not to be judgmental. But as a former food sufferer, I know that the overblown way I thought about food was the root of my problem.

When it comes to seeing the whole truth about what food can and cannot give you, inquiry cuts through the most intractable beliefs or stories. Left unquestioned, beliefs are so powerful that they can keep you bound and suffering for a lifetime. Thankfully, inquiry can go toe to toe with these beliefs because questions trump beliefs.

The most innocent question can create a tiny fracture that crumbles even the most formidable assumptions. When you're unaware of your beliefs, you're their slave. Inquiry forces you to investigate the stories that cause you to reach for food in the first place. By asking, "What story am I in?" you give yourself the ability to unearth the belief that's been running you. Knowledge is power.

When you're thinking longingly about food or about to eat emotionally, ask yourself why. What belief is causing you to reach for food and look to it for something it was never designed to give you? Perhaps your answer will be "I want pleasure now." or "Life is so stressful right now that I want to experience pleasure to get some relief."

The Truth about Emotions

But let's try taking the belief "taste pleasure will relieve my stress" to inquiry. Ask yourself these questions:

1. Is it true that taste pleasure will relieve my stress? (Whether you answer yes or no doesn't matter.)
2. Can you absolutely know that it's true?
3. How do you react when you believe that taste pleasure will relieve your stress?
4. Who would you be without that thought?

Now turn the statement around to its opposite: "Taste pleasure *won't* relieve my stress."

Ask yourself whether the opposite statement could be as true or truer than your original statement.

Come up with three supporting examples to prove the veracity of the opposite statement. Here are some examples:

- *No matter how delicious the food, experiencing a pleasurable taste in my mouth will distract me for only those few seconds that the food is in my mouth. It can't ultimately relieve my stress.*
- *My stress is caused by either a painful belief or by living a lifestyle that's not suited to me. Eating fixes neither.*
- *Overeating pleasure food when I'm not hungry increases, rather than relieves, my stress. If I overeat, not only will I have to contend with the situation or belief that caused the stress, I'll have increased my stress by piling on the guilt, blame or shame that always follows overeating. And I'll have to deal with weight gain, bloating, discomfort and low energy to boot.*

Food, Freedom, and Truth

Practicing inquiry into persistent beliefs, not just once, but repeatedly, weakens the destructive thinking patterns that drive your misalignment with food. Eventually, those patterns disintegrate, freeing you up to have a healthier, more balanced relationship with food.

THE TRUTH ABOUT EMOTIONS

The Role of Emotions in Perpetuating the Illusion

Emotions are like weather. One minute you're enjoying life, reveling in the warmth of a summer day, gazing up at endless blue skies, and the next minute, an ominous wind stirs up the leaves next to your feet and dark thunderclouds roll in. One minute you feel light and happy, the next minute you feel heavy and contracted.

As human beings, we're programmed to seek out pleasure and avoid pain. We don't like negative emotions because they create unpleasant contractions and agitation in our bodies. So it's no wonder that, if food has been your drug of choice, when a negative emotion erupts in your body, your first impulse is to numb out with food.

But the discomfort doesn't stop with the contraction. When a negative emotion hits, you step out of the joy of simply being and identify with the ego, which can make you feel like you're possessed by a crazed demon. Not only does this unseemly creature bring suffering, it actually feeds on it. The minute a negative emotion takes you over, it demands to be fed, and pushes you to create more pain, either for yourself or for others.

Identifying with your ego and a negative emotion causes you to become a pain magnet. You either pick fights with others, provoking them to identify with their own egos, or you stoke your internal emotional fire with more stressful thoughts. With your help, the ego pens an even more painful story of woe than the story that created the emotion in the first place.

The Truth about Emotions

To better understand emotions, let's look at how the ego operates. The ego is a phantom that only exists as the belief "I am a separate entity." Essentially, the "you" that you have come to know yourself as—the ego—is really just a concept: "I am a person, who is separate from you, who believes this, that, or the other thing."

Because the ego is not real, it can't exist in the only place that is real, the timeless present moment. Instead, it uses thoughts and feelings to move you into its unreal, time-bound world of past and future. The ego judges, characterizes, and compares the present moment with its story about past moments, but it can't actually enter and experience the now. And the more dramatic the ego's story, the more the more it demands your attention, keeping you identified as a separate "me." As long as you're paying attention to thoughts and feelings, you're living in an illusory world. From this place, rather than experiencing life directly, you're cut off from natural joy of your true self. This is hell.

Like everything else, the ego wants to exist, to stay alive. It's constantly working to keep you out of the present moment, because it doesn't exist there. With the present moment safely obscured by a thick veil of thoughts and feelings, its survival is assured, and it can go on about its business pretending to commandeer the ship of your life.

Because they manifest powerfully in our bodies, emotions are the ego's most potent illusion-maintaining tools. But, like the ego, they are phantoms—nothing more than painful thoughts that we christened with belief. The ego presents you with stressful thoughts, one after the other, hoping to get your buy-in. As soon as it has it, as soon as you believe a stressful thought, an emotion is born and quickly lodges itself in your body.

Happily, there is a silver lining in this dark cloud of negative emotions. Whenever a negative emotion arises, it's a hopeful sign that you're ready to heal the conditioning that triggered it and gave it life. Somewhere, buried deep within your psyche, lives a core belief that the emotion is signaling you're ready to see through. You do this by shining the light of your consciousness onto it so that it can be released back into that consciousness.

The word "emotion" comes from a Latin root meaning "to move through or out," and when you feel sad or angry or afraid, that emotion is just passing through. Ramana Maharshi, a great South Indian saint said, "What comes and goes is not real." Because emotions and thoughts come and go, ultimately, they are not real. Like everything else in the illusory world of duality and impermanence, emotions don't come to stay. They just pass through, temporarily obscuring the reality of your nature, like a thunderstorm momentarily covering the blue sky.

Holding onto Old Feelings and Generating New Ones

By holding onto old negative feelings and generating new ones, we strengthen our emotional eating habit and lock it in place. Unwittingly, we cling to the past, think about it, and replay our version of whatever painful occurrences we think have happened to us. We choose blame over forgiveness and insist on seeing our version of a story as more important than harmony and peace.

To reverse this, we can realize that we are not actually holding onto the past event. We are holding onto our story about it. Because painful stories never tell the whole truth, they are lies. By believing it you are making this lie more important than your happiness. Once you see that this is what you have been doing and you realize that holding onto is making you suffer, you can begin to let go of the past and stop creating negative emotions about it.

Another way we hold onto old feelings is by reinforcing our negative self-images. We give unpleasant meanings to the things other people say or do, and we project these painful beliefs onto ourselves. For example, when I was a young child, I assumed that a friend of my mother's who was laughing while I was dancing in front of the coffee clatch in the family room as laughing at me. I gave this meaning to her laughter: my dancing was terrible and I was a joke. I created a self-image that there was something terribly wrong with me. I populated this self-image with feelings of shame, embarrassment, and hopelessness. Every time I made a mistake or someone teased me, I allowed that experience to reinforce my negative self-image.

This self-image directed my behavior in all areas of my life. Rather than following my heart, I made choices that kept me safe. Afraid of triggering the shame associated with my self-image of being "a joke," I carefully avoid the spotlight.

My relationships were often train wrecks because of my unconscious reasons for entering them. I chose partners not because I wanted to be with them, but because they accepted me. Desperate to turn myself into what I thought a particular boyfriend wanted, it didn't even occur to me to vet him as a potential partner. Because I wasn't being discriminating, I chose unsuitable people—people who didn't make sense for me. And, because I was entirely focused on changing myself into my partner's ideal, I also lost touch with any sense of an authentic self.

Like so many people, I found myself living a life I didn't like because I unknowingly created structures that didn't support my happiness. I unconsciously chose men who were critical of me and reinforced my negative self-image. I chose a career that was not aligned with my life purpose, doing something that I was neither good at nor enjoyed. Trying to avoid triggering my negative core belief that I was no good led me right back to it again and again. With these two major life structures—relationship and career—out of whack, I found it very difficult to be happy.

Without realizing it, I was generating negative feelings and reinforcing limiting ideas and my negative self-image. I was constantly creating negative feelings and pumping them up with more stories. The stories created new negative beliefs with more painful feelings attached to them. And because I didn't

The Truth about Emotions

know how to deal with those feelings, I ate too much. Understandably, overeating created even more negative beliefs and feelings about myself, reinforcing my original core belief.

I was unhappy because I was acting out of fear all the time. I ignored the trustworthy promptings of my heart in favor of what my ego assured me was the risk-averse path. Ultimately, I discovered that the ego had been lying and that this so-called perfect path was the road to my suffering.

To break the habit of holding onto old feelings and generating new ones, you must realize that you are not actually holding onto the past event, only to your story about it. Painful stories never tell the whole truth, which means they are lies. By believing them, you make the lies more important than your happiness. Once you see that this is what you've been doing and realize that holding onto these stories is making you suffer, The first step in reversing the habit of holding onto old feelings and generate new ones is to see it. This makes it conscious. And then from the wise, compassionate part of you is able to help you see that the pattern doesn't serve you. You'll then be able to notice when you're about to give a negative meaning to something someone said or did, and interrupt it by telling yourself, "Oh that's just conditioning from my past prompting me to interpret her words this way. This time, I won't do that."

If you can see this old habit and realize that there is nothing wrong, you did nothing wrong, you can set the intention to have the awareness to choose differently next time. And if you go unconscious and do it again the next time, simply realize that this pattern of creating and reinforcing conditioning is just part of your programming as a human being. There is no problem here. Then, you can have compassion for yourself about it and recommit to staying conscious the next time. In this way, you set yourself up perfectly for healing.

The Truth about Emotions

Exercise: How to Stop Creating Cravings and Negative Emotions

Close your eyes. Take some deep breaths and just let your body completely relax. Release any tension in your neck, brow, and shoulders.

Imagine that you're boundless space—no beginning and no end. You're omnipresent. Before the earth and planets formed, there was you and when the sun dies, you will still be here. Everything, all worlds, all objects, all beings arise and subside within you.

This body that you have come to think of as you is simply a manifestation of the divine oneness that appears within your spaciousness. You simultaneously animate it and are witness to its comings and goings. As the all-pervasive oneness, you devised this game of separation and this vessel of flesh to enable you to experience yourself. And then you got caught up in the game and confused this body with yourself.

Feelings, thoughts, and sensations arise unbidden within you, the spacious witness and creator of all. From this vantage point of spacespace, notice the stressful thought arising: Life is so hard.

You as consciousness see this thought and decide that it's true. You believe it. You forget all of the times when you felt blessed and life felt effortless. You forget how gratifying it can feel to face challenges and learn and grow, and instead assume that the thin sliver of truth: that "life can feel challenging sometimes" describes the totality of the life experience.

Out of this belief, a merging happens., Yyou identify with and merge with the stressful belief, and a negative emotion is created. You may feel powerless, hopeless, or angry at God or life.

This negative emotion gives rise to a craving. The ego creates dissatisfaction, unhappiness with how life is unfolding and a subsequent desire to have life look and feel different than it does right now. The ego's function is to create dissatisfaction, via thoughts that oppose the present moment. Once this happens, you notice a craving arising, a frantic powerful desire to find and consume pleasure food.

But what if you didn't act on it this time? What if you saw the thought and decided that it wasn't true? You would circumvent the entire negative-emotion-creating process. Without your belief or consent, the thought is powerless. It can't command your attention and no emotion can be generated. This is how you stop creating negative emotions— by noticing a stressful thought and turning away from it when you realize that it's a lie.

The Truth About Life After Inquiry

What do you do after you've debunked the ego? You've depended on it and lived by its counsel for so long that you may feel as if you've been left without any visible means of support—as if you're standing on a high dive on a foggy day, twenty feet up, bouncing anxiously on the end of a narrow board, peering down into opaque whiteness. You can't go back because the fog has swallowed the line of the board behind you, leaving no return pathway or frame of reference. If you decide to throw caution to the wind and fling yourself off the board, what will be there to catch you?

This is where meditation comes in. Rather than excavate the mind as we do in inquiry, in meditation, we bypass it, and land in our true identity, essence. When we're meditating, we can't look to memory or experience for guidance. We take a leap of faith, give up our frame of reference, and choose the unknown over the known. Leaving the familiar land of thoughts, beliefs, and emotions, the domain of mind-dominated consciousness, we become like the explorers of old, sailing into the mystery beyond the horizon.

Ironically, what feels like taking a risk ends up being the easiest, safest choice of all. We step off the diving board to find a safety net right under our feet. In aligning with the silent, present awareness, the nothingness that we melt into in deep meditation, we find our true home. We might imagine that entering the silence will feel foreign, after living caught up in thought, but this joyous, stillness is what we have been all along. We've been so identified with the chatterbox in our head that we never consciously availed ourselves of the nourishing rest of the thought-free state, just below the level of the mind.

Through meditation, we move from our heads to our hearts and allow ourselves to dive headlong into the space between our thoughts—the place where painful thoughts, feelings, and beliefs can't follow. Meditation gives us someplace to land after we've pulled the rug out from under the ego through inquiry. This place is our true nature and no sense pleasure can compete with the joy and satisfaction that comes with living from there. The inner experience of aliveness is where the juice is, where true happiness lies.

Cave of the Heart Meditation

Imagine yourself moving from your head (the ego's world of thoughts, emotions, and cravings) into the space of the heart (the world of your true self). You're floating downward into a delicious, peaceful, joyous space of freedom: the velvety black cave of the heart. It's a restful place of ease, where nothing is required of you, a place free from the stresses and problems of daily life. Simply rest there for 5 to 10 minutes and recharge your batteries. Pick a certain time each day to devote to this practice.

Dis-identifying from Emotions

Taking feelings personally is one of the main ways the ego keeps us identified as a separate "me." The first step in learning how to dis-identify from feelings is to notice them when they arise, rather than taking them personally. But what does it mean to not take a feeling personally?

It means seeing the feeling as one of the many things that are arising in your awareness in a given moment, without attaching to it. For example, here is what is arising in this moment: a car driving by, leaves blowing in the wind, the feeling of keyboard against my fingertips as I type. I don't identify as the leaves or the car or the sensation in my fingertips. I don't merge with them and think that I am them because they register as neutral experience delivered to me by my senses. They don't erupt in my body the way feelings do.

Let's say that anger is also arising in this same moment. Not taking it personally would mean not owning it, not seeing it as different from any other phenomenon that is arising. Anger and leaves blowing in the wind would carry the same weight. Again, this is much easier said than done because it involves moving against our programming. When a negative feeling arises, our natural instinct is to jump in with both feet and *claim it as ours*. We identify with it and merge with it, becoming anger, sadness, or boredom embodied. We believe that it's our anger and as such, we feel justified in expressing it and acting it out, usually to the detriment of our relationships.

When a feeling takes us over, we literally lose ourselves in it. We lose our connection with our true self and forget that we are spiritual beings. Instead, we get duped into believing that we are something we have never been, the ego. Following our programming, we become the feeling, losing all objectivity, and we feel powerless to do anything but react to it.

People talk about feeling overwhelmed by a feeling or a craving. This is perfect description of what happens when we become identified with our feelings. Our power comes from creating some distance from them and moving back into awareness.

Thankfully, this is easier than it sounds. To do this, first notice that a feeling is on the scene. You can say to yourself, "A craving is on the scene." This noticing and labeling begins to extract you from the clutches of the feeling. Then, take it one step further by saying to yourself, "Oh that's just a craving; it's not me. I'm over here noticing it. And if I'm noticing it, I can't be it." This immediately cuts the power of the feeling and allows you to experience some objectivity and relief. From this place, it's much easier to use whatever tool you choose to dismantle the conditioning that gave rise to the feeling in the first place: inquiry, allowing the feeling to be present, or simply moving back into alignment with essence via meditation.

The Challenge Posed by Negative Emotions

Once we know how to dis-identify with feelings, we might feel like we're totally equipped to face anger, stress, fear, sadness, and worry. But these emotions pose our most formidable challenges. Why would we expect our new tool to be a match for them when our healthy habits haven't had time to take root?

That's the ego for you, always demanding perfection. We have the tool—why shouldn't we be able to use it flawlessly? I'll tell you why: five hundred gazillion prior experiences of reaching for food to soothe ourselves at the tiniest hint of a negative emotion. We've spent years reinforcing the habit of innocently comforting ourselves with food.

So and now we expect ourselves not to salivate when the bell rings.

It's like asking a one year old who is taking her first steps to run a marathon! Yet the ego castigates us if we falter. So of course, new out of the box, we expect ourselves to be able to effortlessly create a new habit, lifting ourselves out of our past behavior, out of the well-worn path of the known and the comfortable and into the "new." We expect perfection in the face of perhaps the most difficult challenge we face in becoming free from our eating addiction.

We forget that this is our growing edge. We forget that we have no map, no experience in this new direction that we're carving out for ourselves. It's like asking raging floodwaters to change direction because we hold up our hands and yell, "Stop." Now isn't that a wee bit unfair for the ego to expect?

It isit's important that you be gentle and patient with yourself as you take steps to heal this pattern. Avoid setting yourself up and writing off this new healing process as "one more thing I tried and failed at." Healing can and will happen, with plenty of tolerance, intention, patience, and practice. These are the qualities and behaviors that we need to form any new habit. And the more you reinforce your new habit of dis-identifying with feelings, the easier it will be to follow it the next time a negative emotion arises.

Disappointment and Food

Disappointment is a natural part of life. Yet in the ego's movie script, the scenes involving disappointment all get cut. The ego assures us that if we follow its plan, life will deliver the unbroken happiness we expect. The ego's movie contains only sunny, cloudless days and we convince ourselves that if we only follow the ego's directions, we can live a charmed life.

However, when the inevitable and happens and life deviates from the ego's plan, even in a small way, the belief arises that such a thing shouldn't be happening. If we order our eggs over easy, for example, and the server delivers them scrambled, we get upset because that shouldn't have happened. After all, we made our preference clear. How could life, in the form of a communication snafu, have had the audacity not to conform to our expectation? But eggs are nothing compared with not getting the promotion we've been working toward for years, or not being loved by the one we love, or watching our closest friend get sick or, God forbid, die.

We all know that, in spite of our most painstaking efforts and scrupulous planning, life does always not cooperate and conform to our desires. We work hard in school and go to college, and after graduation, we can't find a job. Or we take great care of our health, eat well and exercise our whole life, and we still contract a terminal illness.

Then, there's the other kind of disappointment, the kind we experience when we follow our desires and see them realized in ways that are beyond anything we ever expected, yet still don't feel fulfilled or happy. Then what?

When disappointment rolls in like a dark cloud obscuring our natural happiness, what are we to do other than follow the course of least resistance and reach for food? This is a loving impulse on our part. We try to soothe ourselves by distracting ourselves from the true cause of our discomfort: our uninvestigated thinking.

What could be more natural? We grew up in a culture that used food to distract us from life's discomforts and unpleasantness. When we were children and the nurse gave us a shot at the doctor's office, she rewarded us with a lollipop. It's how we've been conditioned. Rather than learning to stay with and experience painful sensations, we're taught to switch into a more pleasant experience as quickly as possible. It's no wonder that at as grown-ups we reach for a cookie or a cocktail or jump into a new relationship to replace our lost lover when we feel disappointed.

The problem is that the cookie provides only a few seconds of a pleasurable taste sensation in your mouth. When the sensation disappears, you have to refill your mouth with another bite, then another, and on and on. Before you know it, you're shoveling and stuffing, two-fisted if necessary, just to keep reality out of your awareness.

If you tell yourself the truth, though, cookies really can't help you escape your disappointment. Here's why: The cookies taste so delicious that it's hard to stop eating them. But you're so distracted by the "should" and "shouldn't" thoughts underlying your disappointment that after the first few bites, the taste hardly matters. You're too busy shoveling in cookies and thinking and feeling to notice the taste sensation that you hoped would distract you from the discomfort of feeling your disappointment in the first place.

The feeling of disappointment the cookies were meant to numb then grows into something that dwarfs the original

Food, Freedom, and Truth

feeling. Not only do you have the original disappointment to contend with, you now have bloat, low energy, possible weight gain, shame, blame, self-castigation, and low self-esteem piled on top of it. The truth is that food never solves the problem, and it adds to it significantly. Yes, in the moment, it distracts you with a nice taste, but then what? It's hard to stop eating pleasure food once you have started, and after your party with food ends, you feel worse about yourself than when you were only dealing with your original disappointment.

This is the truth about food and disappointment. In fact, this is the truth about using food to distract yourself from any emotion. Food wasn't designed to do this for us. Whenever you look to food to give you something that it was never designed to provide, you add to your burden and cause yourself more suffering. This realization is key to breaking the cycle of emotional eating.

How do you stop turning to food when you experience disappointment? Practice. Set the intention to keep seeing the whole truth of food, rather than only appreciating it for its taste appeal, and ev, we can break the cycle. In the past we've been in denial allowing the ego to lure us with the promise of a few seconds of delicious taste in our mouths. But once we've consistently remembered the to see the whole picture, we can't be fooled by the sliver of truth that the ego shows us. Eventually, you will be able to interrupt the automatic feeding impulse and break the emotional eating habit for good.

Rewriting the Scene

When an emotional eating attack happens, the impulse to reach for food can be powerful. We go unconscious so quickly that it can be difficult to choose to do something else that doesn't involve eating. In those moments, the rest of the world disappears and we become the craving.

Because we have strengthened and reinforced our habit of reaching for food when an emotion is on the scene over many years, forming a new habit means first creating a template for change in our consciousness. We have to first believe that change is possible before we can step into the role of our new self who no longer eats emotionally. This can be challenging if you have no frame of reference for being with emotions that doesn't involve trying to avoid them through food.

Our imaginations can be a great help in creating a new template for change. Athletes know the power of visualizing a successful performance ahead of time. Prior to a game, many athletes imagine themselves "in the zone," playing the game of their lives, and they are far more likely to play well during the actual game.

Exercise: Visualization

Close your eyes and imagine your last emotional eating attack. Allow the movie to play in your head. What just happened? What are you doing or saying? What is your internal conversation about what is happening? What are you telling yourself about what is going on? What are you feeling and needing in the moment?

Now, imagine a different scenario. Watch yourself start to open the refrigerator or pantry. Look down, see your arm reaching, and stop. Watch as you interrupt your habitual pattern and, instead, walk out of the kitchen. Next, ask yourself what you're feeling and what you need in this moment. Imagine giving yourself what you need, whether it's acceptance, appreciation, or love. Whatever it is, imagine giving that to yourself, now.

Alternatively, ask yourself if you're aware of something greater in yourself, something that doesn't need anything, that is already happy and enjoying even this feeling of desperation or craving? Here is a hint: it's that which is looking out from your eyes. If you can get in touch with this "something else," put your attention there. This feeling of "happy for no reason" is who you really are, the spiritual being that doesn't need anything and is perfectly content with whatever is happening. Explore this connection with the being that witnesses the emotional upheaval from a distance.

Now, if the feeling is still present, imagine yourself allowing it to be present and at the same drop any story about it. If you notice yourself feeding the emotion with more stressful thoughts, simply stop and move back into the sensation of the feeling. Inwardly welcome it and tell it that it has your full permission to be there for as long as it needs to be.

The next time an uncomfortable emotion arises, practice welcoming it and allowing it to be present. If you eat emotionally, it's no problem. Simply rewrite the scene and imagine giving yourself what you need in that moment, or shift into identification with the part of you that has never needed anything. Then, invite any residual feelings to remain for as long as they need to be present.

In this way, you create a new habit of tolerating feelings and giving yourself what you really need by dis-identifying with feelings altogether and moving back into essence.

Taking Responsibility for Creating Your Feelings

The spiritual component of healing emotional eating involves taking responsibility for creating your feelings and responding to them when they erupt. When you're aligned with the ego and believe untrue, stressful thoughts about life, food, and yourself, those beliefs give rise to actions and choices that undermine your happiness.

Most of us aren't masochistic, yet unwittingly, due to our programming and mistaken beliefs, we behave in ways that are contrary to our own well-being. For example, if we misunderstand life and doubt its benevolence, we let fear overtake us, and may end up taking a job that doesn't fit for us just because it means a stable paycheck. Then, when we're unhappy because we're spending most of our time doing work that we don't like, we try to get happy through food.

When we question our painful, mistaken beliefs, we discover that believing them has made us suffer, and led us to behave in ways that caused us to suffer even more. Seeing this enables us wake up out of the ego and rest in our true identity, essence. When we really examine this pattern, we move in the opposite direction and align with our true self, stop creating negative emotions, and make choices that support our health and well-being.

From this new place of inner peace and contentment, our choices and actions support our happiness. When we live in this way, we're joyous and engaged in life. Consequently, we don't have to reach for food to try to be happy. We live life with the awareness of our true identity as a spiritual being.

What choices will you make from re-aligned with your true self—as a spiritual being encased in flesh? Who knows how your life will unfold. One thing is certain—your willingness to be open to this spiritual perspective about yourself and food means that you are at a very exciting crossroads in your life!

How to Stop Creating Negative Feelings

If you were to write a job description for the ego, it would begin as follows: engaged in the primary business of creating negative feelings and self-images. Not surprisingly, the ego, wishing to avoid the ranks of the unemployed, tries to thwart any attempt to dismantle its feeling creation machine. Let's look at how the machine operates.

A negative thought arises and we have a choice to either believe it or not. The ego keeps presenting us with thoughts until it gets our "buy in." Essentially, it's asking us, "How about this one, do you believe it? No? What about this one?" It keeps throwing negative thoughts against the wall until one sticks. When we believe a negative thought, even a little bit, the ego throws another one our way. Assuming we cooperate and take the bait, pretty soon, we have a full-blown unhappy story.

Most negative feelings are born out of self-righteousness— hence the expression "righteous anger." Like a prosecutor building a case, the ego creates a most compelling story, encouraging us to feel entitled to whatever resistant feeling arises. As we believe each line, it becomes evidence supporting a negative feeling's right to exist. If we have a litany of reasons justifying our perspective, we start believing justified in our perspective. We're right, other people are wrong, and the payoff is that we get to feel superior. Then, quicker than you can say "I got triggered," a feeling erupts, and we can puff out our chests and say, "Forget love, relationship, or practicality, I have a right to feel the way I feel."

The Truth about Emotions

On the flip side, the feeling that arises feels so real and true that we think, "Wow. Look at how I'm feeling. I must be right in believing my thoughts about this situation. Even though the ego got what it wanted—creating a negative feeling so that we would feel separate and contracted, it doesn't stop there. It tries to blow the feeling up even more by feeding it with more stories.

How do we interrupt this pattern and disable the ego's feeling creation machine? For one thing, we have to set the intention to stop creating negative feelings. There is a certain energy that comes with creating negative feelings that can be addictive, so it's important to go inside and ask if you really want to stop this. If the answer is "yes," begin by asking for help and setting the intention to intercept negative feelings before they erupt in your awareness.

Because the human feeling generation machine is designed to swing into action instantaneously, to interrupt it, and stop creating negative feelings, you must more awareness to your stressful thoughts. As soon as you recognize that a stressful thought is on the scene, intercept it by not merging with it.

What do I mean by that? We're programmed to believe negative thoughts and immediately identify or merge with them. To avoid this, catch the thought before it turns into a belief by noticing it and choosing not to believe it. Once you believe the thought, it becomes much more difficult to avoid creating a negative feeling. At this point, you can still cut the feeling off at the pass by noticing that you just bought into a thought and saying to yourself, "Wait a minute, I just noticed that I am believing this thought. But, is that even true?"

As soon as you see the ways in which the thought doesn't tell the whole truth, you're home free. Congratulations! You've just thrown a monkey wrench into the feeling generation machinery and prevented a feeling from being formed.

Depression, Repression and Living Your Life Purpose

If you're binging or eating compulsively, you're repressing your feelings. Often we repress our feelings when we're afraid to stand up for ourselves. You might be thinking that people won't like you or your spouse will leave you if you start speaking your truth, saying "no" when you mean "no," or asking for what you want. The first step in learning how to speak my truth was acknowledging that people's anger couldn't physically hurt me. I was safe. Next, I realized that even though eating could delay and blunt my reaction, it didn't serve me. When I stuffed my feelings with food, not only would I beat myself up, take my upset out on those around me in passive aggressive ways, I repressed my feelings.

Depression is a repression of life that happens when we avoid saying what we need to say and doing what our hearts are guiding us to do. Rather than being assertive and taking action in our lives, we feel stuck and depressed about it. When we feel powerless and unsatisfied in our lives, and if turning to food for comfort has been your habit, it's no wonder you are repressing your feelings and eating compulsively.

If you have a pattern of repressing emotions, this can leave you feeling hopeless and depressed. You might be repressing your feelings or feeling depressed if you aren't living your life purpose because you're listening to and following your negative thoughts instead, a pattern that will lead straight to the refrigerator.

Other reasons that you might feel depressed are because you're out of the flow of life, not resting enough, or making

Food, Freedom, and Truth

enough time to do things that feed your soul. If you are busy *doing* all the time, you won't be able to slow down and get quiet enough to listen to your intuition. Life communicates its intention for us, our life purpose through our intuition. When we spend time every day in essence, we are able to feel the gentle prodding of our intuition, which guides us in the direction of fulfilling our life purpose. But if we're frantically *doing* all the time and not giving ourselves enough downtime, we'll miss its insights. Living your life purpose means doing things you enjoy and are good at. You know when you're aligned with your life purpose because you feel happy and excited about what you're doing.

Exercise – How to Stop Repressing

Make an intention for yourself to stop repressing your feelings. Then, ask to be shown the backlog of emotions that you have been repressing. There is an undercurrent of negative emotion that exists just below your conscious awareness. When something happens to trigger these emotions, you find yourself feeling out of control and eating compulsively. Asking to be shown what you're repressing and setting the intention to allow yourself to feel rather than express or repress your feelings, will break this pattern.

Soon after you set this intention, be prepared for insights to arise. Then, record whatever fearful beliefs come up and take them to inquiry. In addition, speaking from your heart by asking for what you want and saying "no" when you mean "no," will also help to break your repression habit.

Food, Freedom, and Truth

Sadness: The One Exception

Unlike other negative emotions that come from the ego and cause you to feel bad by disconnecting you from your inner wellspring of happiness, there is a kind of deep sadness that comes from essence. While it's true that the ego is often creates sadness by encouraging us to be chronically dissatisfied over our lot in life. The knee jerk human reaction is to resist whatever shows up. It's a "glass half empty" way of looking at life that can stem from an underlying belief like "life is unfair" or "Others get what they want, but I never do." This sadness can be a surface feeling, hiding a deeper layer of anger.

Although the payoff of such beliefs may be feeling justified and self-righteous about the unfairness of it all, we still suffer over our conclusion about life and others. As a "have not," we experience being separate and disconnected from all of the "haves."

On the other hand, the sadness that comes from essence is the result of choices that created a life that doesn't fit for you. If you're feeling this deeper sadness, it comes from living a life where you spend most of your time doing things that you either don't like or aren't good at. How did this happen? In your life up to this point, rather than moving toward joy, you often listened to and followed the fearful voice in your head, instead. "You can't do that, what would other people think?" "There's no money in being an artist, how will you pay your bills if you do that?" "You'll regret it later, if you don't have children."

Egoic choices put security first and cause you to move away from what you came here to learn and experience. You did this out of self-love, innocently hoping to shield yourself from future pain. But the result has been just the opposite because cultural conditioning tends to come from the ego. Whether it comes to you as advice from others who claim to be wise and know what is best for you or as examples of others who appeared to suffer either by not making the safe choice or thrive by making the safe choice, it always leads you away from your own wisdom and living your life purpose. In this way it causes to you feel disconnected from your heart, which leads to emotional eating.

Following the subtle promptings of your heart, moment to moment, is intrinsically joyful. They will never steer you wrong. Realizing that it's not up to you to determine the course of your life is such a relief! Thankfully, there is something far wiser than your mind guiding your life and when you tap into it, trust it, and act from it, life becomes easier and more joyful. Human evolution is designed such that we often learn by suffering, that life is about surrendering, not steering.

The gift of this deeper sadness from essence is a clue that something is off in how we've been living. If we continue to make choices from fear, our suffering grows more intense. At a certain point, most people connect the dots and make changes that align them with essence and their life purpose.

Feelings: Good, Bad, or Ugly?

In and of themselves, feelings aren't good or bad, or helpful or unhelpful—it's what we do with them that counts. If anger arises and does its dance, you might experience an urge to eat, if that is your habit. Yet, if you let yourself feel the anger and use it as an opportunity to inquire either into how you're living and communicating, or into the beliefs that created the anger, then it can be helpful, then it can serve your growth.

A feeling is red flag, an indication that you believed a stressful thought. But the opportunity inherent in a feeling is less about the feeling itself and more about what you do with it. For example, if boredom arises you could inquire into how you're spending your time and get motivated to find something else to do that's not boring. If fear arises, you may want to ask yourself, "What is the worst that could happen if what I fear could happen, actually happens?" Making the fear more concrete usually has the effect of showing that its worst manifestation is not so terrible and cutting the power of the belief that gave rise to it.

If sadness is present, there is the possibility that it can motivate you to do things that moves you out of the sadness. But unless you ask yourself, "What do I need to do to get out of this sadness?" or "What is this sadness about?" the sadness doesn't get you anywhere.

Sadness can also point you to a belief you have that is stopping you from doing something you would love to do, something that would make your heart sing. Maybe there is something missing in your life that you need to explore. If this is the case and you use the sadness as an impetus to inquire, the sadness is helpful.

For most people, when a feeling arises, it triggers an impulse to distract themselves—through eating, watching television, getting busy, or shopping. In the moment of following those impulses, the feeling has no value. Not only that, the impulse to distract can lead to a pattern of habitual avoidance through unhelpful behaviors.

Instead, if you can break out of this cycle and use the discomfort of the feeling to prompt you to inquire then you have given it a purpose. Asking yourself the following kinds of questions, allows you to make the best use of feelings: "What am I believing that is causing me to feel this way?" "Is there a misunderstanding or a mistaken belief that I need to question?" "Is there something I need to address in this moment or in my life?" Even if you follow the impulse to distract yourself from the feeling, all is not lost. It's never too late to inquire.

Connecting with Your Inner Child to Heal Conditioning

Inner child work is a powerful tool for healing conditioning because it connects you directly with the building blocks of subconscious memories. Working with a therapist who does inner child work or a hypnotherapist, can help you to release the deep conditioning blocking your daily experience of freedom and happiness.

The reason inner child work has the capacity to heal deep subconscious wounds is that we store childhood memories in the form of images. It's not the painful event itself that causes the conclusions that make up our core beliefs, but rather these images. If we work with our imagination to replace the wounding images with new positive, nurturing images through inner child work, we can release the negative conclusions we formed about ourselves and life that continue to cause suffering.

Recently, after a painful breakup, I conjured up an image of myself as a child and asked (internally) what this little girl needed. As I gazed at her, she regressed to little more than a year old. Ordinarily I would have asked her how she was and what her life was like. However because she was too young to be very verbal, I connected with her visually instead.

She looked up at me as if to say, "Please pick me up now." I lifted her and she placed her little curly head on my shoulder. I could feel her body shutter. She began to sob softly. At one point, I started to set her down and she held onto my hair as if to plead with me not to put her down.

Food, Freedom, and Truth

Then, I asked to see an image showing me both how I had been damaged as a child and the conclusion that I drew as a result of it. I saw myself as this very young child, playing alone in my playpen for hours. My mother on the scene somewhere but not connected to me. I felt invisible, as if I didn't exist for her.

No wonder my inner child didn't want me to set her down. She felt orphaned, completely alone, and unloved. I told her that she never had to be alone again. I was there for her and would keep holding her as long as she wanted me to. For days on end, I continued to carry her with me. At one point, when I felt that she was ready, I finally set her down, assuring her that I would continue to check on her to make sure she was okay and hold her whenever she wanted me to.

Then, it came to me, the core belief that had caused my relationship based suffering was this, "If I love people, they will reject me." There was no doubt that this was my core belief because just thinking it unleashed a flood of tears. When you uncover a core belief, it will certainly be attached to strong emotions.

Soon afterward discovering this core belief, I saw the string of men I had fallen in love with. I remembered how with each one, I had always felt a sense of impending doom about the relationship. Something inside me believed that as soon as I gave my heart to a man, the relationship could never work out because he would find a reason to reject me. And right on cue, they always did.

My need to have men whom I loved, love me back was so strong because I was looking for a way to invalidate the core belief: If I loved them, they would reject me. Ironically, sensing my neediness was probably the thing that caused my boyfriends to run in the opposite direction, turning that belief into a self-fulfilling prophecy.

As I replayed each relationship and its aftermath in my imagination, I saw that whenever I was jilted, I would fantasize longingly about sexual aspect of the relationship. It occurred to me that perhaps the reason I did this was because I had never bonded physically with my mother. I was using relationship to fill that void and supply the touching I never received as a child. It was almost as if I was imprinting on these men, the way baby animals imprinted on their mothers. The wounded child in me was using their touch to heal this deep wound in my psyche.

Next, I asked to be shown the sub-beliefs attached to the core belief: If I love someone, he will reject me. Here the list I came up with:

- I'm unlovable,
- I'm hopelessly flawed,
- I should never have been born,
- I can't make it on my own,
- I will never be happy,
- God is playing a cruel joke on me,
- I need someone else to love me to survive.

To begin to heal this complex, I took each of these beliefs to inquiry. Please recognize that uprooting a deep-seated complex like this requires vigilance. It's likely that I will need to stay connected my little girl and keep giving her what she needs for quite some time. In addition, to fully heal this complex, I will likely need to take each of these sub-beliefs to inquiry many, many times.

Exercise – Inner Child Healing

Find a private place, close your eyes, relax, and ask to be directed to the place of your deepest wounding. Be patient and soon an image of yourself as child in a particular situation will surface. Ask your child about herself. What does it feel like to be her? How does she experience her life? Now, ask your child what negative conclusion she drew about others, life, and herself based on this experience. This negative conclusion is the core belief at the center of the psychic complex that has been sapping the joy out of your life.

Then, ask your child what he or she needs from you to heal the wounding. Imagine yourself offering it to her. For the next several days, each evening, before you go to bed, check in with your child and continue the healing. If something happens during the day to upset you or hurt your feelings, check in with your child. In your imagination, offer her whatever comforting she needs, assuring her of your love and intention to always be there.

Next, ask to be shown the cost of carrying this belief. How have you lived your life as a result of holding onto it? Asked to be shown images of the situations that triggered and reinforced this painful belief. To heal the whole string of experiences, imagine giving these past "yous" what you needed in those situations.

The final step in your healing is to neutralize the complex that has grown up around your core belief. To do this, you have to first make it conscious, just like you did with the core belief that spawned it. With pen in hand, jot down any other related beliefs that come to mind. Using this stream of consciousness approach, map out the complex. Finally, take the original damaging belief as well as the sub-beliefs in that complex with the strongest charge to inquiry. Continue practicing inquiry until those beliefs are weakened to the point that you no longer believe them. You can know that you no longer believe them when they no longer carrying an emotional charge.

Inner Child Meditation for Emotional Eating

Find a comfortable private place, where you can sit for a few minutes without interruption. Close your eyes, take a few deep breaths, and relax. Using your imagination travel back to the time when you first formed your emotional bond with food. What was happening in your life? See this child, not getting what she needed and feel her pain. Then watch as she reaches for food to fill the hole in her soul. What is she telling herself about life, the adults in her world, or her own worth as a person? What conclusions did she come to?

Look into her eyes and see the pain there. Let her know how sorry you're that the adults in her life can't be there to protect her and take care of her and make her feel loved. Let her know that you're there for her now. Ask her what she is feeling and what she needs from you. Say, "I love you and I'm here for you? What do you need from me right now? What can I say or do? What can I give you? Feel your heart move out to her and envelop her in your love. Give her what she needs in this moment. Look at her. What is happening? How does her face look? Look into her eyes, what do you see? Let the healing that is happening radiate out into your own heart. Feel the empty place in your soul that you have been filling up with food, fill up with pure love and joy.

Embrace this child and tell her that you love her and that you will never leave her again. The bond between you is unbreakable. From today forward, you will always be there for her and will check in on her regularly. Whenever you feel the urge to reach for food and you're not hungry and it's not time to eat, you will connect with her. By asking her what she is feeling and needing, you be confirming for yourself that up until now, your emotional eating habit was your way of trying to fill an emotional need with food. Food not only can't fill the need, it actually makes you feel worse, emotionally, physically, and spiritually. Instead, you will ask your inner child what she needs in this moment and offer her the love, reassurance, appreciation, that represents her true craving.

THE TRUTH ABOUT BODIES

Making Peace with Your Body

For years I used to suffer over how my body looked. If I weighed five pounds more than my ideal weight, I couldn't be happy. I couldn't enjoy friends, family, work, or creative pursuits because I was fixated on this area of perceived imperfection. It made no difference to me that others didn't notice much less object to the added weight, I knew it was there and that was all that mattered.

Unbeknownst to me, I was programming my discomfort into my subconscious, by what I chose to pay attention to. I hadn't learned the fundamental governing principle of life in a human body: pain is unavoidable, but suffering is optional. All suffering is internally generated. I didn't know then that my happiness less to do with external events and everything to do with the attention I gave my negative thoughts about those external events and circumstances.

In other words, my discomfort about my so-called imperfect body had nothing to do with the fit of my jeans or the number on the bathroom scale. Yet, innocently, I created my unhappiness by telling myself the story that my inability to maintain my ideal weight meant that I was irreparably flawed and would never be able to achieve my dreams.

How do we stop perseverating about doughy midsections or lumpy thighs? How do we stop being miserable about how we look? Realizing that this suffering is self-inflicted, caused entirely by believing your negative thoughts about your body, how do you think about it? What do you do to reinforce that thinking and keep it going?

Food, Freedom, and Truth

You might counter that we live in a society that is completely obsessed with youth and beauty. How can we be expected to ignore its influence when everyone around us is caught up in it? While it's true that we are bombarded by images that reinforce culturally sanctioned ideals about bodies, in order for them to impact us we still have to buy into the ideas about the importance of external appearance. You can choose to suffer or not.

Whenever you're feeling bad about how you look or anything at all, the most powerful question you can ask yourself is, "What am I telling myself to cause myself to feel bad?" What is your negative self-talk? Uncover that.

Next, look at your behaviors. What are you doing to reinforce your negative body image? How much time do you spend staring at yourself in the mirror examining your physical flaws? If so, what do you say to yourself while you're standing there? Are you busy appreciating all of your best physical features or are you tearing your body down? If it's the former, this negative self-talk is reinforcing your negative self-image.

The reason dis-identifying with the image in the mirror is not as easy as it sounds is that over the years, you've reinforced the habit of creating an emotional connection with it. Understand this and be gentle with yourself as you create a new relationship with your body, one rooted in functionality rather than a two dimensional image.

Perhaps you do other things that reinforce your negative self-image like looking at pictures of models in magazines or watching entertainment television. Do you watch shows that glorify physical beauty? You can keep doing these things, but understand they come with a cost: reinforcing the culture's superficial values and perspective about bodies.

The Truth about Bodies

How do we avoid suffering over how we look? Begin by accepting the fact that this is the way your body looks right now, in this moment. This is the way it's now, at least until you take steps to change its appearance by losing weight or getting more fit. Can you change the way your body looks in this moment? Of course not—it's too late. The moment has already passed. You don't have to like it, but think about it. Isn't it completely irrational to suffer over something that you can never change?

If your belly protrudes over your waistband or your thighs rub together when you walk, you might have a thought like, "It feels bad to be in my body at this weight." But this is just a thought. It's a story. Many people have bodies with the same characteristics and their bodies don't feel bad to all of them.

If you believe that it does feel bad to everyone, where is your proof? Have you interviewed every overweight person? It's just the way the body is right now. That's just what it does. What's bad about that? If you believe the story, "it feels bad," that's how you create your suffering. "It feels bad" morphs into "I don't like it. It shouldn't be there." to "I hate this." Hating it's arguing with and resisting reality.

You don't have to believe the story, "my rolls of flesh feel good" or "my cellulite is beautiful," because these are just more beliefs. You don't have to tell any story about yourself or your body. If you want to stop suffering over how your body looks and feels or anything else, for that matter, all you have to do is ignore your negative thoughts.

If the thought "cellulite is ugly" appears in the mind, notice that that is your cultural conditioning around fat. It doesn't have to cause you to suffer if you simply see it as conditioning rather than the truth. Notice it and don't touch it. Just leave it alone. It doesn't matter. Then do whatever it takes to counteract that thought. Maybe cellulite is beautiful can counteract that thought, but usually positive affirmations that are the exact opposite of what you actually believe don't work because you don't actually believe them. Belief is the elixir that gives power to a thought. Otherwise it disappears like writing on water.

Have you ever tried to make yourself like something you don't like? How did that work? You can't really force yourself to like something you don't like. Perhaps this is why trying to make myself believe that "My cellulite is beautiful" never would have worked with me. I'm not saying that it can't work for other people. Perhaps it can. But because I haven't vetted it in my own experience, I can't teach it.

If you want to use the mind to counteract or neutralize the mind, try something like, "It doesn't matter." "It's not who I am." It's not important." "It doesn't make me a bad person." "It doesn't mean anything about me." "It doesn't make me less attractive or less valuable." "This doesn't have to ruin my life." You can focus on being beautiful on the inside, being kind to others, being a good person, and living a good life. That's what's important. These thoughts are perhaps more believable to most of us that the thought, "cellulite is beautiful." The bottom line is that if you're overweight find a way to be okay with that for now. It's always just for now because you might lose weight tomorrow.

If there are people who label and judge you based on your cellulite, does it really matter? Know that this is their conditioning, their egoic mind. If they are judging you, they are certainly judging themselves. Have compassion for them because they are caught up in the same suffering and pain that has been plaguing you. The difference is you're learning to get beyond it.

Simply understand conditioning for what it's. It's not the truth. If others believe their conditioning and reject you for it, it's a shame. But you can't do anything about it. You can only change your own thoughts, not how other people respond to you.

Maybe you'll lose weight tomorrow but for now, why create suffering over the size of your body. It's a waste of time and energy and doesn't help you lose weight. If beating yourself up helped you lose weight, then everyone would be skinny. It doesn't do any good, so why create more suffering for yourself?

If you're overweight, for as long as your body continues to appear that way, make an effort to ignore your negative thoughts about it so you don't suffer. It's not an attractive state to be suffering over how you look and not liking yourself. That demeanor can impact other aspects of your life. If you're busy hating yourself thinking, "I'm sure you're judging me too" how is that going to impact your relationships or your career choices?

We have all known overweight people who have been beautiful inside and out, like Queen Latifah. Seek out other examples like hers and remind yourself of them, when you feel bad. Remembering them will undermine the critic and weaken your negative conditioning about your body. It does this by reinforcing the whole truth: you're far too great to ever be reduced to any negative idea about your external appearance. It's possible to have an imperfect body, one that the culture shuns, and lead a completely happy and fulfilled life.

Wanting the Perfect Body

Wanting a perfect body, as the culture tells us we should is a particularly painful egoic desire generated by the critic. The critic tries to convince us that unless we have the perfect body, we won't make it in life, we won't get the things we need to be happy. Yet, the truth is *we already are that happiness,* and any impulse to look for it outside ourselves is misguided, futile, and causes suffering.

This doesn't mean you shouldn't ever want to lose weight. If you're overweight, essence intends us to bring the body back to a healthy size. This is natural. Yet this natural impulse toward health is easily coopted by the ego—the critic and the dreamer. Suffering comes into the picture from all the conclusions and projections we pin onto losing weight, like the belief that losing weight will bring happiness and success. It's the "happily ever after" aspect of our fantasies that keeps us hooked.

Believing that we need the body to look a certain way is how the ego tricks us and keeps us searching in the wrong direction for satisfaction and happiness. Wanting a different body in this moment is like wanting the sky to rain candy canes. This moment can never be any different than it's, and *the body that is appearing in this moment can never be different.* It's too late—the moment has passed—it's over, and we're onto a different moment. Freedom comes from accepting this moment as it's. This body is manifesting in this way right now, and from that place of accepting the body as it's appearing right now (not forever—but for right now), a shift is possible.

The Truth about Bodies

Suffering over our desire for a different body doesn't fulfill that desire; it doesn't change our body. Because it makes us miserable and doesn't change anything, it's completely irrational! Seeing the truth of this connection between resisting what our body looks like right now and suffering can help us see that resistance is a waste of energy. It's futile and just makes us feel bad.

We grow by seeing the truth and living in a way that is congruent with it. Our new wisdom aligns us more and more with essence and makes us less likely to fall victim to the ego's tricks. Once we accept our body as it's right now, then we are free to choose to change it, but from a balanced, rather than a deluded place. This is the battle: resistance versus acceptance; the ego versus essence; self-delusion versus the evolutionary impulse for Truth.

The Desire to Lose Weight

As you wake up out of your ego and learn to stop listening to the voice in your head, you come more into balance with life and your body. Out if this movement can come the intention for a healthy body.

You can instantly know whether and impulse comes from essence or ego depending on how it feels. Intuitions from essence are subtle and the message is loving and kind and promotes health and balance. The ego, on the other hand, conveys its overblown desires loudly, through thought. Unconcerned with health or balance, the ego wants to be admired. It wants to be the most beautiful and special so that it can stand above the crowd.

If your body is overweight, the desire to lose weight can come from either ego or essence. If the desire comes from essence, it's a gentle impulse that honors the body and intends its health and wellbeing. There is no blame or self-castigation, no sergeant barking orders at your newly formed weight loss boot camp. Essence doesn't cajole you or try to lure you in by creating a romantic story about how wonderful life will feel after the weight loss. These tactics all belong to the ego's weight loss plan.

If your desire to lose weight comes from the ego, there is no problem with this. Just notice it and tell yourself the truth about it. Ask yourself if you can know that the romantic stories that the dreamer is weaving about how wonderful life in your new svelte body will be are true. Can you really know how life post weight loss will look? Can you really know how weight loss will impact your life? If you're beating yourself up about how your body looks now, take a moment to honor yourself. Feel compassion for yourself and all that you've been through in your life. Being human is no easy feat and no one's life is easy. Weight loss is not like a Zamboni for your life, smoothing away all of the bumpy difficulties and challenges in your path.

The Body: Amend or Transcend

Overweight bodies and what to do about them can be a polarizing topic. In the mainstream, overweight is considered an epidemic, a problem that our country needs to solve. In the mainstream, people lament the personal and societal devastation it causes siting a plethora of physical, emotional, and economic implications. Yet, in many spiritual circles, the shape and condition of the body is irrelevant. After all, we're spiritual beings having a human experience, not the other way around. So the question is what do you do if you want to become self-realized and your body is heavy, try to make it smaller or loosen your identification with it. Amend it or transcend it?

Everyone is different and no answer from the outside will uncover what is best suited for you. If you have a spiritual orientation, you might say, "wait a minute, I know that my path is to move out of identification with the body altogether, so I might as well take the path of transcendence." While it may ultimately be true that eventually, we all are released from body identification, yet if you move to this place prematurely, without inquiring into what is uniquely true for your evolution, you may miss an opportunity for growth that is a better fit. Everyone's path is different. Don't preclude the possibility that you may need to lose weight before you can love yourself and be at ease.

"But if I do that, aren't I just playing into the hands of the ego, and giving into desire," you query. Yet if you get quiet, align with essence, and find that you're being moved to change your exterior, there is wisdom in it. By creating a more positive exterior, you transform your interior simultaneously by unseating an unconscious, negative self-image related to be being overweight that's keeping you from experiencing the freedom and joy of your true nature.

No formula for healing body image issues works for everyone. Some people need to get a slimmer body in order to be at peace with it. While other people feel moved to transcend identification with the body altogether. The key question is which approach, amending or transcending the body, is life moving you toward? To get a true answer, and by that I mean *your answer*, requires you to move out of your ego, get quiet, and align with your own inner wisdom.

Aligning with essence requires making peace with your body by either accepting its current appearance. First, you accept the truth of the way your body looks right now. Although you may not like the appearance of your body, there is no denying that it looks the way it looks right now. Acknowledging the truth in this way aligns you with essence, the seat of your inner wisdom. From here, you can discover what, if anything you're moved to do about your weight.

If your body is heavy, chances are you're carrying around a negative body image that is blocking you from getting thin. This self-image sabotages your actions because beliefs, emotions, and desires impel action. If you hold a mental image of yourself as fat and you create an identity around it based on the belief that who you're is fat, you will create that reality by eating too much.

All negative self-images are self-perpetuating and a self-image of being fat is no exception. When you have an identity of being a fat person and you view being fat as a negative characteristic, the ego will work like mad to keep that limiting and painful self-image in place. In other words it's job security for the ego. The ego creates the problem, suffers over it, and then encourages you to eat to feel better.

If you believe that who you're is fat, you will unconsciously behave in ways that hold this image in place. You see yourself as fat, so you will eat more, particularly of the high taste, high fat foods that created your overweight in the first place. This negative self-image of being fat causes you to feel bad and feeling bad moves you to eat pleasure food to help yourself feel better. You eat a lot, gain weight, feel bad about it, and eat again. It's an insidious, self-perpetuating cycle.

To counteract the ego's tendency to maintain its self-images, you have two choices. You can either throw out all images by using inquiry to debunking the "I am the body" assumption, or you can replace your negative body image with a positive one.

To neutralize this image, every time you think of yourself as fat, replace that mental image of the fat you with a mental image of yourself sporting a trimmer body. Because images go right to the subconscious, inspiring pictures can be great tools to reprogram our negative beliefs.

See if you can find pictures of bodies, your body or someone else's, that you find beautiful and tape them up around your house. If you don't want others to see them, tape them to the inside closets, lay them inside your drawers, or put them in your wallet. You may scoff at the idea of creating a vision board and populating it with either pictures of a thinner you or pictures of bodies you admire, but if it can help you to heal conditioning, why not try it?

Without realizing it, while trying to lose weight, I was actually reprogramming my negative image of being overweight. I did this in two ways: by avoiding mirrors and by only wearing loose fitting clothes. My rationale was that both mirrors and tight clothes reminded me that my body had grown past my liking, and those reminders hurt!

When I didn't feel my clothes binding my body, when I didn't see a heavier face and body reflected back to me in the mirror, I felt thinner, not to mention happier and more comfortable.

A few years earlier, I'd lost weight before and all of my clothes felt loose. This tactile memory reinforced the self-image that I was thin, even though I hadn't yet reached my goal weight. And without the reinforcement of the mirror, I reduced my exposure to evidence of my heavy body. You could say that I was deluding myself and running away from the truth and you would be right on both counts. But there was method to my madness. Essentially, my strategy was: fake it till you make it—and it worked for me.

When you'ren't reminded about the size of your body, by seeing it or feeling it, you don't think about it and you don't suffer over it. When you'ren't thinking about being fat, does it bother you? All of our suffering stems from attaching to our thoughts.

Remarkably, with a thin-self image created by my loose clothes, I behaved like a thin person. I ate healthy and I ate less. If I had thought of it, I could have taped pictures to the refrigerator of a thinner me or of my head on top of Christy Brinkley's body.

If you're body is heavy, chances are you carrying around an image of yourself as heavy. Imagining the possibility that you could look different can neutralize the negative images that you're holding in your mind. Using pictures, whether they are

Food, Freedom, and Truth

physical or mental, can help motivate you to create a thinner body, if that is what you want.

Whether you want to change your body to create a better self-image and feel better about yourself or whether you want to transcend the whole game of trying to look better, there is benefit. Neither approach is right or better or more spiritually evolved. Whichever path you choose opens the door to growth and healing deeply imbedded conditioning.

The Antidote to a Negative Body Image

When you see yourself as fat, often that is all that you see. You miss all of your other virtues and talents. Just like the pleasure seeking child hooks us with the thin sliver of truth about eating pleasure food—it tastes good, and leaves out the whole picture of the shame, blame, weight gain, bloating that we also experience when we eat, the relentless critic hooks us with a slim sliver of truth about our identity—our apparent physicality, and ignores the immense totality of what we are–divine, vast beyond measure, ageless, and deathless. We are unique manifestations of the wholeness, with qualities and talents that will never be matched or duplicated ever again!

The critic's assessment of our worth only looks at the spare tire around our middle or the new wrinkle and doesn't include the beauty of our compassion, generosity, or kindness. It only values the outer and keeps us stuck in the ego's superficial worldview—our physical appearance is the only thing that other's value about us. It says, "Forget about ever being happy unless you're young, thin, and beautiful. After all, do you see images of old, ugly, fat people in magazines, or on television, or in movies?" "There's your proof," the critic will tell you. "People don't want to look at you if you're old, ugly, or fat, not if they have a choice anyway." If that's how you look, you will become invisible, nobody.

Take a moment and investigate how the ego's negative self-talk about your body contributes to a negative, painful self-image. What do you tell yourself as a result of having a body that you don't like? How does this self-image impact how you live? How does it hold you back? You might be surprised to discover the full extent of its impact in your life. Seeing the truth about this creates a powerful incentive to shift out of your negative self-image.

Although it may be true that some people may be attracted to you initially based on your outer appearance, but they fall in love with your heart. How long do you remain under the spell of people's outer beauty, if they are ugly on the inside? Isn't it true that if there is little to love about how they move in the world and treat others, the magic of their attractiveness loses its power? They literally start to look ugly. On the flip side, if people are plain on the outside and exude an inner radiance because they are comfortable in their own skin and treat others with love and respect, they start to appear more attractive on the outside.

Exercise – Transforming a Negative Body Image by Focusing on Your Virtues

Take out your journal and make a list of your positive inner qualities. Today, if a negative thought about your body arises, replace it with a positive thought about an inner virtue. Then, reread your list. Tonight before you go to bed, reread your list again. And over the next week, add to your list and reread it daily. Pretty soon, when a negative thought about your body arises, it will be second nature to dismiss it, and see the whole truth of your beautiful soul.

Perfection

Chasing perfection is one of the critic's favorite games. It hooks us with the promise of an imagined future of everlasting happiness, if only we follow its program of creating the best possible "me." Yet, even if we achieve some of the goals in the ego's perfection scheme, life never feels as we hoped it would. It never feels completely satisfying.

The ego uses perfection to keep itself employed. Coyly assuming that if we stay focused on striving toward an idealized future, it hopes that we will forget to notice what's already here. Ask yourself, "Is there something that's here right now that requires no effort to experience and is happy already?" "Happy for no reason" is our birthright. It's always available to us and when we're quiet, when we stop thinking, we experience it.

The question, "Is something here, right now, that is happy already?" can transport us out of the false, fantasy world into the reality of the present moment. The key to moving back to reality is in the act of noticing. The minute we notice that we're paying attention to and following our thoughts, we are back in awareness and out of the egoic mind.

Striving for perfection, on the other hand, keeps the ego employed and keeps us living in a false, mental world. As long as we are caught up in in a concept like perfection, we're lost to ourselves, wanting to come home but traversing a path that points us in the opposite direction.

The ego thinks we need to have it all together to be happy. It imagines a future moment when we "arrive," when the years of work that we've done on ourselves finally pay off, and our dream of a "perfect me" living a perfect life manifests. To get from our current flawed "me" to the glorious realization of a "perfect me," according to the ego, we have to be vigilant, tyrannizing ourselves every time our humanness shows up. In other words, if we don't eat the way we planned or if our body doesn't look just so, we castigate ourselves and make ourselves miserable.

If we overeat or eat junk food one day, we think we've blown it, and tell ourselves that after all we've done and tried, we're nowhere with this issue. Healing from eating and weight issues that took a lifetime to develop is possible. I'm living proof. But it doesn't happen overnight. Progress happens, plateaus, seems to be undone, and then moves forward again. The cliché of moving two steps forward and one step back has certainly been true for me.

Yet to be healed, we don't have to get everything right and we don't even have to get to someplace called "100% healed." Perhaps we believe this so the ego can tell the story "I'm 100% healed or look how perfect my eating or my body is now." The salient question is: Is how I'm eating right now or is the size of my body negatively impacting my health? If not, let it go. Why torment yourself? Ask yourself: Is okay for me to be human? Is it okay to be imperfect?

If you're answer is no, you're setting yourself up to be miserable because the truth is there's no such thing as a perfect person. Certain people appear to have it all together but can we really know their experience? Can we know what their life feels like? Everyone's life has built in challenges. Imagine how boring it would be if it didn't. Challenges seem to be part of the plan. Otherwise, how would we grow? Would you really want

Food, Freedom, and Truth

to live in a world without challenges or growth? Sounds like a pretty boring existence to me!

One of those challenges for those of us who aspire to be perfect is learning to love and accept our human foibles, our imperfections. For us, the question is: can we be tender with ourselves when we don't meet our expectations for ourselves? Knowing that life isn't easy, can we learn to be tolerant and loving toward ourselves? At least, if we're going to perfect something, why not perfect being kind inside? Why not perfect accepting ourselves especially when we let ourselves down or don't meet our expectations?

The other issue with chasing perfection is: transforming ourselves into our ideal of what a person should be keeps us locked up in the illusion of a separate personal identity. No matter how wonderful you become as a person, it's that very concept of personhood that our evolution is waking us up from! Chasing perfection is literally like moving deck chairs around on the Titanic. No matter what you do, the ship is going down. No matter how perfect your character becomes, life's evolutionary impulse is leading you toward self-realization, seeing that you never were this person you're playing at.

You're something infinitely greater. Uncanny as it may sound, the person who feels like you is appearing in the vastness of who you really are. Each character is flawed and yet each has an important role to play in the evolution of the oneness. The imperfections and foibles as well as the talents and skills of your particular "me," the whole package that comprises your character, serves the whole.

The Truth about Bodies

Body Image

Our culture values youth and looking good disproportionately and most women in particular expend tremendous time and effort trying to measure up. Inundated with images of young, thin, beautiful people, it's natural to assume that you should look that way too.

Rather than concocting a plan to eliminate the young, thin, and beautiful among us, or cursing our lookist culture, it's helpful to understand how you contribute to your suffering over how you look. It's not enough for the culture to tell you to look a certain way; you have to *believe* it. You do it to yourself by buying into the story that you have to look perfect forever to lead a happy, successful life.

The answer to this messy predicament is simple: finding a wise relationship with your body, one that you don't suffer over. But how the heck do you accomplish that when images of perfection are everywhere? Not only is it possible, you can create that relationship, right now and experience it in any moment.

Close your eyes. Imagine how it would feel to *not* suffer over how your body looks. "Hold on just a minute," you say. "You mean to tell me that I can stop suffering over how my body looks, just like that?" I know it sounds like a tall order once you realize that how you think about your body has been the source of endless suffering! But the bottom line is: yes you can. The trick is shifting your perspective.

If you can relate to the body from your own innate wisdom, rather than from ego, you can sidestep your body identified suffering. The most important thing is to move the notion of body from an intellectual understanding and into the direct experience of the "beingness" that you're. From that place of being, you see the body for what it's, a useful tool, a servant, a vehicle.

A healthy alignment with the body is an inner experience of your true nature and realizing that who you really are has nothing to do with your body. When you believe you're your body, you're always at risk because the body ages, gets sick, and dies. When you think you're it, you see yourself as vulnerable and frail. But from the direct experience of beingness, you're the witness of the body, watching whatever happens to it from a place of fond detachment.

Take a moment to experience your beingness. What does it feel like to look out from your eyes? We are accustomed to identifying with the appearance of the body and imagining how others perceive it, and we forget that *we are that which is looking and experiencing everything*, rather than what is seen. What does it feel like to be the seer rather than the seen?

When you move into the experience of being by feeling the aliveness in your body or moving back into that which is looking out from your eyes, the role of your body falls into its right relationship. When you practice this you get taste of how essence sees the body. From essence, your body is beautiful, useful, and loved for those things rather than who you are.

From the ego, your body's appearance is the basis for all sorts of overblown stories. "Having a body this size means I won't be loved, I won't ever be happy." essence, on the other hand, doesn't need job security. It's who we are so we can't fire it! From essence, the body appears the way it does and you're grateful that it functions. Yes, your body is different from someone else's body and that's okay. It's not important. From essence, your body's appearance has nothing to do with you're lovability. You're precious no matter what. Essence is like an unconditional loving parent, delighting in you no matter what you say or do or look like.

The ego has another shtick altogether. To it, the body is all about appearances. It has an image of how it's supposed to look and if it doesn't match up to that image, it causes you to suffer over what that means about you and your potential for happiness in the future. If your body doesn't measure up, you're inferior or weak or undisciplined and your life will never work out the way you had hoped. Thankfully, all painful stories, including the story that you tell yourself about appearance are false.

From essence, there's no story telling. There's just appreciation, a love for the body because it functions, is useful, and gives you experience of being human. Dis-identifying from the body means seeing the difference between how the ego treats the body and how essence treats the body. When you're identified with the body, you're ego is treating the body in a way that's not loving. Essence doesn't do that.

From essence there's no comparison. Essence doesn't say, "His body looks better than mine or wow I wish I could look like that in a bikini." Notice how the mind's always comparing bodies. "My body should be this way and it's not." Whenever you compare, you're in the ego, looking at the body.

When there's no comparison, but a simple looking out from the eyes, there's just a seeing of the vehicle that the body is. It's just as it's, with no judgment or characterization. There's just noticing, "This is how this body looks now."

The bottom line is that focusing on outer beauty is suffering. So why would you choose that? When you're at the check out line at the supermarket and you see the magazines with bikini-clad women on the covers, notice how they play right into the ego's body identification and it's need for your body to look good relative to other bodies. So don't look at them. Instead, say something kind to the cashier. Be in the moment as the loving being that you're looking out of your eyes, recognizing that ego is in the magazines.

The ego can be everywhere around you, in others and rampant in the culture, but if you're coming from essence, you'll bring that out for someone else. You can serve others by putting your attention on being essence, even when they are aligned with their egos, to help them connect with their own essence.

Exercise – Dis-identification with the Body

Here are some steps to take to help you begin to dis-identify from your body:

1. Practice experiencing your beingness. Get intimate with what is looking out from your eyes, the experience of seeing rather than identifying with the seen.

2. Stop looking in the mirror or at least make looking in the mirror a very quick experience. Just do what you need to do and move on. They say, " the devil is in the details?" In this case " the ego is in the mirror." The ego, through its "Critic" sub-personality, uses the mirror as a platform to tell you all the things that are wrong with your body. You can choose not to give it this opportunity by not spending a long time looking in the mirror.

3. When you see your body and other bodies, notice where your noticing is coming from. Are you noticing from ego or from essence? When comparison and judgment are present, "you know who" is also present and that's where your seeing coming from. Luckily, the very act of noticing that you're coming from ego plunks you right back in essence. It's as simple as acknowledging, "Oh that's just the ego prattling on," and ignoring it. Because the minute you buy into one thought, it has another one waiting for you. Pretty soon it's written a novella and dumped you right into a mind-created hell world.

Food, Freedom, and Truth

Armed with these three steps you have the tools to experience the body in a whole new way, the way the wise part of you or essence has always known it. Thankfully, you can begin to honor and appreciate its service, rather than bemoan its warts. You can marvel at it as consciousness itself as well as the vehicle in which consciousness manifests. In this way, you wake up out of body identified egoic hell. Good luck with creating the new habit of experiencing your beingness in each moment!

Change the Lenses of your Glasses

While talking to some friends at a party, you happen to glance over to see an exquisite creature sashaying through the door. Every feature is perfection. Her face and body look as if Michelangelo himself sculpted the contours. Your mind immediately activates the critic. In a few short seconds, your self-esteem falls down around your ankles. Then dreamer clamors to get into the act and you move into fantasy. "If only I looked that way she does, then my life would be a paradise. When I walk into a room, every head would turn, and men would line up begging to date me.

Beauty moves us into essence when we let it. Yet, when beauty manifests itself through another human form, it can trigger a fear response. Rather than seeing the truth, that who we are animates every form, we categorize the person as other, believing that we are inadequate and lacking in comparison. Assuming that relationship and happiness are finite resources, reserved for the genetically fortunate few and because we don't think we measure up, we hang our heads, slink away, and resign ourselves to a fate of living pedestrian, uneventful lives.

The other underlying assumption in the ego's hypothesis is that other people value only our outer appearance. Many of us fantasize about walking into a room and all eyes instantly land on us. It's true that people can be temporarily taken in by outer beauty and perhaps for some, being with someone whose outer appearance is pleasing is enough for them.

Yet, for most people, inner beauty is not enough to create and sustain a loving connection. Sometimes, when a vision of loveliness floats in, she opens her mouth, and a river of ugliness flows out. Nothing has changed on the outside, yet we can no longer see her as beautiful in the same way.

On the flip side, we love to be around plain looking people, who radiate a beautiful presence. Amazingly, their inner beauty begins to transform their outward appearance. Pretty soon we see their inner beauty first and value that much more than how they look on the outside. In The old expression, "beauty is as beauty does," shows us the whole truth of beauty is that beauty is really about our beautiful inner qualities shining through.

Many of us see being loved as a key to happiness. Our cultural obsession with outer beauty stems from believing that if we look good, others will love us and want to be with us. But love is who we are through and through, whether we fit into our skinny jeans or not. The more we are connected with essence, our inner source, the more this love radiates from our presence, and the more others want to be around us.

Ironically, it's this outward flow of love from our own hearts that enables us to feel love. What a blessing to realize that, contrary to our romantic ideas, we don't need others to love us to feel loved. Whenever we want to feel loved, we simply focus our attention on loving others and serving them. This releases the river of love inside of us.

If you're valuing yourself solely based on how you look, realize that you're doing this and make a conscious choice to change the lenses of your glasses. See the deepest truth of who you're by experiencing that which is *looking out* from your eyes, rather than what you see in the mirror. This radiance is what people fall in love with about you. From this vantage point everyone is beautiful.

I Robot

Your body is your robot, your earth-exploring vehicle. As spiritual beings, in order to have a physical experience on planet earth you need a robot. Just like I need a computer to be able to make my thoughts visible to others, we need our robots to see and operate through. If your goal is to wake up out of your programming, into the realization of your true nature, a human body is your ticket to play. A dog body or a guppy body just won't cut it.

The confounding thing about body-minds is that once we have them, we get very attached, so much so that we actually begin thinking that we *are* our body-minds. Yet, just because need bodies to be able to move on the physical plane and have the experiences we need to evolve and deepen in love, it doesn't mean that represent the totality of who we are. In other words, we don't have to identify with them.

The healthiest attitude to have toward your body is to see it as a beloved servant, the temple of the soul. Honor it, respect it, and do your part to keep it healthy by feeding it healthy food, exercising it, and giving it enough rest. Other than that, there is nothing else you need to do.

How it looks is none of your business. How much did you have to do with determining its eye, skin, or hair color? Did you "spec out" this body and design it as if you were created a work of art? Of course not. You simply got what you got.

When your car battery dies or your computer is running slowly, you don't take it personally. You don't think you're your car or computer and feel inferior because they are not running optimally. Similarly, why would you take it personally if your robot get sick or loses its hair? It's not you.

Food, Freedom, and Truth

If you're doing the basics to keep your robot healthy, how it ages is none of your business either. Your body is doing its job by taking you where you need to go and allowing you to have the experiences you need to grow and evolve. Becoming overly focused on creating a good looking body, so that other body-minds will admire it or using it's weaknesses to manipulate others or get attention or sympathy, all of these motives come from the ego.

Ideally, from the ego's perspective, it wants the body to beautiful and forever young to help it get the money, fame, success, security, and partner it wants. Without these things, it assures you, happiness and security are not possible. Yet, as essence, you naturally want to care of this robot body that has been entrusted to you. You don't see it as you, just something life has generously put at your service, to live through and experience from.

THE TRUTH ABOUT ENDING EMOTIONAL EATING

Changing Perception is the Key to Transformation

Tobacco consumption wasn't reduced through regulation or legislation, but by changing how people perceived the cigarettes. The public view of smoking changed from, "I want to buy cigarettes because smoking is glamorous and sexy. And it will make me more popular and give me more status." to, "This is a deadly, disgusting product. Not only don't I want to smoke, but I want to be far, far away from people who do smoke"

In the same way, healing your malignment with food completely, rather than superficially, means changing how you view it and changing your life, if it's unfullfilling or out of balance. If you romanticize food by imbuing it with the power to make you feal good, you activate your egoic mind and produce a craving. If, on the other hand, you look at it and say, "I know that would taste good but ultimately, if I eat it, I will feel worse. Not only will I have to contend with the situation that triggered me and caused me to reach for food, but I will have to deal with the shame, blame, self-castigation, bloat and potential weight gain that comes from overeating pleasure food."

If you relate to food in this way, using the mature, rational part of yourself, your ego isn't activated. Aligning with essence enables you to percieve the whole truth about what food can and cannot give you.

If you view food as anything other than nice taste nutrition, essence encourages you to look deeper. Is it really true that

The Truth about Emotional Eating

food can make you happy when you areyou're sad? Is it really true that food, can comfort you or be your friend? Can it really numb you out for more than a few moments and protect you from having to deal with your feelings or your problems?

To heal completely, you have to disempower food by seeing it clearly and removing your romantic projections and by filling the hole in your soul that caused you to seek pleasure and distract yourself through food. You see the food in the context of its true function, rather than in the misguided role you have given it. In this way, you change how you view food and ultimately heal your food addiction.

Relationship with Thoughts

When one of my teachers said to me, "Laura, your mind is not your friend," it turned my world upside down. Up until that point, I had always believed that *I was my mind*, and the thoughts that cropped up inside my head were my thoughts. And if I wasn't doing all of this thinking then, who was?

Up until that moment, I assumed that the thoughts that were appearing in my consciousness were my own private affair, in the same way that I was not privy to other people thoughts. I could be chatting with people, and for all they knew I was having the time of my life. But on the inside, I was bored out of my tree, thinking uncharitable thoughts about them. And since these were my private thoughts that I believed I created, they couldn't harm any one else.

However, this new information from my teacher confused me and caused me to question so many assumptions about life. I was quite sure that thoughts arising in my awareness couldn't impact anyone else. Other than that, I was completely befuddled. If these weren't my thoughts, then whom did they belong to? And if I wasn't my mind, then who was I?

My teacher's comment implied that even though my thoughts couldn't impact others, they might be harming me. I had to know, how these thoughts that had been masquerading as me, were not my friend.

Donning my sleuth's cap, I began monitoring my thoughts. I soon learned that most of them are negative and arise unbidden. When I gave these negative thoughts my attention and christened them with belief, I saw that I suffered. Although we are programmed to pay attention to thoughts, we do have a

The Truth about Emotional Eating

choice. We can simply notice that a particular thought is on the scene and turn away from it. It's our attention and belief in thoughts that give them their power.

If someone told you that from this moment forward you would have to live without 99% of your thoughts, you might panic. But if you actually tried it, you would quickly discover that you really don't need most of your thoughts. In fact, without them, your life proceeds quite beautifully—actually feeling better to you than before. The reason for this is a little known yet powerful law that governs our human experience: *our happiness is directly proportional to the extent to which we are able to ignore our minds.* Consequently, the wisest possible relationship we can have with our egoic thoughts is to ignore them.

Most thoughts come from the ego and only rarely from essence. When you think you're your mind and allow your thinking to direct your life, your life will feel empty and disconnected. If, on the other hand, you turn the reins of your life over to essence and allow it to direct you, you will be aligned with your life purpose. Because essence will always move you toward doing what you came here to do, your life will feel happy, full, and satisfying.

When used properly, the mind is a useful tool. If you can allow the impulses and insights from essence to guide you through life, rather than the thoughts that come from the mind, and only go to the functional mind to perform mental tasks, you will be using the mind using it as it was designed and you won't suffer.

Exercise – Ignoring Thoughts

Today, when you notice that you're caught up in thinking and there is no practical reason for it, turn away from your thoughts and engage directly in sensory experience. In other words, focus instead on what you're smelling, seeing, working on, hearing, or feeling. If you need to use the mind to perform a mental function, by all means, do so. Otherwise, practice turning away from thought.

Where's the Benefit?

When something happens that you didn't anticipate or don't like, do you notice your hand reaching for food? Or do you ask yourself, "What good can come of this turn of events? Does it bring a new opportunity for growth? Can I bust a misperception or glean a truth that I'd overlooked? Even though this situation doesn't fit my picture of what I thought I wanted, how can I use it to create more freedom and happiness?

Every apparent misfortune brings a gift. Life is here to serve our freedom and help us learn to become more loving. If we can see life from this vantage point and look for benefit and opportunity in every circumstance, not only will we be happier, but if this is our habit, eventually we will shift out of egoic consciousness and abide in our natural state of freedom and joy.

Our main job as spiritual beings masquerading as human beings is to pay attention and see beyond apparent inconveniences and setbacks. Once we shift back into awareness, and get curious about what is happening rather than judging it, new insights arise, and we are in a position to harvest these precious opportunities.

Native Americans traditionally used every part of the animals they hunted. They waste nothing. Make this your philosophy about how to approach your life. As you live each day, waste nothing. Each experience is a new opportunity to grow, deepen in love, and let go of what you're not (the false self or ego). If you're unhappy with how life is unfolding, it means that you haven't yet seen the opportunity or benefit.

Often, we don't see how we benefit from a challenging life experience until much later. In hindsight, you realize that if you had been able to do what you wanted to do at the time, you never would have developed a particular quality in yourself. If that so-called "bad" thing hadn't happened, you wouldn't have developed the fortitude and courage to ignore the cautionary opinions of others and risk following your dream. If the guy you thought was "the one" hadn't rejected you, you never would have met your current partner.

When an inconvenient situation arises and it doesn't fit in with your plans, take a moment to contemplate. What benefit could come from this situation? What gift does it have to offer? How can I learn and grow and deepen in love from allowing myself to open to this new possibility and experience it fully? You will be amazed by what you discover!

Exercise – Where is the Benefit

Think of a situation that you currently view as unfair or unpleasant. Take out your journal and list all of the benefits of that situation. What gifts has it brought you or could it potentially bring you if you chose to see it differently?

Your Achilles Heels

Everyone who has a challenging relationship with food and body weight has certain Achilles heel situations that trigger food cravings. The mere prospect of being seated next to Aunt Millie, walking by the break room at work or attending the annual school potluck dinner, with its mile long dessert table, can leave you in a cold sweat.

How can you deal with these challenging circumstances without eating your way through them? Try this exercise to help you come up with some strategies for your Achilles heel situations.

Exercise - Dealing with Achilles Heal Situations

1. Start by telling yourself the truth. Become aware of the circumstances, situations, and people who have triggered your overeating in the past. When you don't know your triggers, you're a sitting duck, just waiting helplessly for the next food disaster to strike. Then, before you know what hit you, you find yourself writhing in pain with an overstuffed belly. In short, becoming aware of your eating triggers keeps you from being blindsided by your Achilles heels.

2. Next, make a list of your Achilles heels. Think of yourself as a general creating a battle plan. Rule number one of warfare is: knowing your enemy. When you make a list you can't pretend that you were caught off guard. And when life takes an unexpected turn and you're caught off guard, you will be in much better shape than you otherwise would have been. You will have created strategies for the situations and people on your list that can be adapted and come to your aid.

Avoid stressful situations. You don't need to accept every invitation that comes your way. Even Emily Post won't fault you for a gracious decline. Don't worry. I'm not suggesting you change jobs because Bill from the mailroom makes popcorn every day, but rather that you look at your life and ask yourself how you can take better care of yourself and make your days less stressful and more enjoyable.

3. Create a plan for Achilles people and situations. If you decide not to change a stressful situation, create a plan that makes it easier to manage. If the prospect of seeing Aunt Millie at the family reunion that you really do want to attend makes

you want dive head first into a container of double chocolate fudge ice cream, plan some social strategies that help you from getting cornered by her.

4. As for the office challenges, take your coffee break at popcorn time, to avoid the most potent popcorn smell. Walk the long way to the restroom to avoid going past the lunchroom to avoid seeing the latest cache of goodies. Make a plan to leave the school potluck right after the dinner portion. Or decide ahead of time that you will allow yourself one small plate of dessert and stick to your plan. Or decide to skip dessert altogether.

5. Create a plan for trigger foods. If freshly baked chocolate chip cookies turn you into a wild banshee then don't offer to bake them for your kids or the bake sale. It's natural that certain foods that were designed for taste, designed make us overeat them, would trigger out of control eating. If you can't moderate them, either give them up for good or create a strategy you can stick to that enables you to stay in control. For example, Wednesday might be dessert night. You don't keep sweets in the house, but every Wednesday night you go out for a hot fudge sundae or cannoli.

6. Finally, remember that the past is not a reliable predictor of the future. In the past, just because the appearance of an Achilles heel meant letting the pleasure seeking child have the upper hand, doesn't mean that you can't change that dynamic now that you have the proper tools.

The Truth about Emotional Eating

It's also important to realize that Achilles heels are the toughest situations you will confront, so don't expect yourself to be perfect out of the box. If you fall into old patterns, see them as opportunities to practice being kind to yourself. Eventually your intention toward health and balance will prevail. It can't be otherwise.

The desire to heal conditioning and become free comes from essence, our true self. The plan is for each of us to become more loving toward ourselves and others. Healing addictions is one of the most loving things we can do for ourselves. Please honor and appreciate yourself for having maturity and courage to follow this pure intention from essence.

Stressful Thoughts and Emotional Eating

Frenzied emotional eating is unconscious and automatic. Because you're not present, it can feel like you need an exorcist rather than a therapist to help you come back to yourself. Cleverly, the ego causes you to go unconscious when we eat emotionally because it knows that there's a way in which you haven't completely committed to overeating junk. On one level, you feel ambivalent about using food to fill an emotional need because the wise part of you knows that it's a poor strategy, one that not only doesn't resolve your emotional discomfort, but causes more suffering down the road!

To heal emotional eating, realize that when you want food and you're not hungry, you're engaged in a fictitious mental story caused by believing your stressful thoughts. In other words, in this moment, you believe something negative about life, others, or yourself. Making this pattern of telling yourself a negative story conscious is a huge achievement because as soon as it happens, you're no longer in the story. Then, from a place of awareness, you can step back and ask whether the stressful thoughts underneath your uncomfortable feelings are true.

All stressful thoughts are untrue, not just those related to abstaining from certain foods. The way to stop suffering is to see that your stressful thoughts are causing your suffering, and in seeing this, it becomes much easier to ignore them.

Just because feelings and thoughts enter our awareness, doesn't mean we have to believe them or act on them—we can just notice them. Being aware of thoughts and feelings rather

The Truth about Emotional Eating

than identifying with and acting on them is a huge leap forward in making peace with eating, weight, and our bodies.

Being Okay With Where We Are

So much of our overeating and eating the wrong foods has to do with not being okay having the experience we are having. Perhaps movies and fairy tales have done a number on us, indoctrinating us into believe life should always feel like a party. But may be they got it wrong and that's not part of the plan at all.

There is great benefit that comes to us even when life doesn't feel pleasant. We grow from every tear we shed, from every moment of suffering, from every time we let life's challenges get the best of us and lose it. And yet there is a way that we can cause ourselves unnecessary suffering. If we suffer over our suffering we add to our burden because we believe that we should somehow know better. After all we have read and done, we should be more spiritual than that.

If we can allow ourselves to just be where we are, feel however we feel, do whatever is in front ourselves to do, rather than comparing our life to someone else's life or to a fictitious idea of what we think our life is supposed to look like, we will be less likely to reach for food. If we can just be where we are right now, we won't need to create the negative emotions that result from fighting with life. Creating fewer negative emotions means fewer trips to the refrigerator.

And if we do happen to create negative emotions, can we be okay with that? Can we let that be and not beat ourselves up over it? Life is a messy business and not easy for anyone. In the face of this reality, can we give ourselves permission to be imperfect human beings grappling with difficult challenges? Can we be okay with where we are? And when aren't okay with where we are, can we tell ourselves the truth about it and be okay with that too?

Living As A Human Being Meditation

Close your eyes and connect with the feeling of aliveness inside your body.

As you go about your day, focus on experiencing your beingness. By all means perform tasks, but see if you can remain connected to that feeling of aliveness in your body. Rather than thinking about what your are doing, enter the experience totally. Become the driving or the cooking or the getting dressed. So often we split ourselves by doing one thing and thinking about another. Today, focus on living life from the direct experience of the aliveness of your inner body. Connect to whatever you're doing using your senses rather than your thinking mind. This is what it means to be a human being rather than a human doing.

The Fun Factor

Lusting after food is lusting after pleasure. When we're looking for a party in our mouths, it's because life feels like anything but a party. Most of us don't let ourselves have enough just plain fun and as a result, we find ourselves sprinting to the fridge in hot pursuit of leftover pizza or coffee almond fudge ice cream, trying to squeeze out a few moments of pleasure by tasting something good.

As adults, we're conditioned to believe that we "should" be responsible all the time. The operative word is "should." We "should" ourselves out of all of life's goodness. We don't have to be saving the world every minute. It's really okay to just take a break and enjoy ourselves, without food of course. Every action doesn't have to be purposeful. Instead, let your job become, making sure you have fun every day. In fact, put it in your calendar!

If you're giving up your current egoic relationship with food, going to food for comfort to avoid feeling unpleasant feelings, you need a new relationship with something else to replace it. Where will you find comfort, pleasure, and relief? How do you do this? It's simple. You find other fulfilling, fun activities that don't involve eating. In this way, you begin to spend more time feeding your soul and form a relationship with something that's always available to you and infinitely more satisfying—your true self.

We're always being fed from our deepest self. Recognizing and acknowledging this helps us to heal and grow. When an unpleasant emotion arises, notice it, allow it to be, and then ask to receive insights and healing. Ultimately, freedom from any issues we have around food is about becoming more

The Truth about Emotional Eating

established in our your true self. To do that, we need to be quiet and not be in a lifestyle that's so busy and stressful that we're constantly getting lost in thoughts, emotions, and doing.

If you're not physically hungry, but feel the urge to experience some pleasure from food, and you don't want to follow that urge, you can move into the heart. Try this exercise:

Food, Freedom, and Truth

> **Exercise – Moving From Your Head to Your Heart**
>
> Imagine yourself moving from your head (the ego's world of thoughts, emotions, and cravings) into the space of the heart (the world of Your true self). You're floating downward into a delicious, peaceful, joyous space of freedom: the velvety black cave of the heart. It's a restful place of ease, where nothing is required of you, a place free from the stresses and problems of daily life. Simply rest there for 5-10 minutes and recharge your batteries. Pick a certain time each day to devote to this practice.
>
> As you practice moving from your head and into your heart, you will weaken your cravings by strengthening your connection to your true self. The more you practice, the more it will become second nature to rest in the cave of the heart during your day.

Junk Food for the Mind

If you ever questioned whether most of what we see in the mass media caters to the ego, notice how you feel after a long session of television watching. Pay attention next time and experience the impact for yourself. Do you feel energized or listless, and empty? If you're like me, you feel drained and it's hard to summon the energy to do something that you would ultimately find more satisfying.

But there is another important reason to curb your television habit. In addition to feeling empty, feeding on mental junk food takes a spiritual toll. The more time you spend watching certain kinds of programs, the more you strengthen the ego's sub-personalities: the child, the critic, and the dreamer.

Many television programs and commercials act out the values of the ego: immediate gratification, youth, physical beauty, money, success, possessions, and fame. Their example sends the message that these things lead to happiness and if you don't have them, you had better create a plan to get them. Otherwise, you might as well hang it up and crawl under a rock. You're doomed to live a life of misery and isolation.

Watch a television commercial and you enter the fantasy world of the pleasure-seeking child. If life isn't providing the enjoyment you're looking for, you don't have the right stuff, so go out and get it for yourself. You deserve it. You need to taste this luscious, mouth watering chocolate truffle right now. You need to own these shoes right now. You need to start drinking this brand of beer right now. If you don't get these things, you will suffer, living in the hellish world of an unsatisfied craving.

Food, Freedom, and Truth

If you want to experience the critic's perspective on life, reality shows and talent competitions are your tickets. You might not have felt at liberty to express your true feelings when our demanding boss piled on more work to your already burdensome load. Yet in the backbiting world of reality television, you're in the comfort of your own living room while others engage in clever insults and fault-finding repartee. Here blame, judgment, and criticism reign supreme and whoever comes up with the most abusive verbiage is the most skilled competitor. Your inner critic can vicariously rant, get red faced, and waive its fists, with no collateral damage to your job.

Diet commercials that show before and after pictures of a success story are the realm of the dreamer. The dreamer is the sub-personality that focuses on the future. Its signature phrase is: if only. If only you go on this diet, you could look great and have a happy life. The advertiser hooks this aspect of the ego, hoping that you will identify with the before image and project yourself into an imagined future of what you could look like when you buy their product. You too, could have a fabulous new physique.

The trouble with exposing ourselves to these images and not so subtle messages is that they feed into and strengthen the ego by validating its worldview. You can say, "I just watch it, but I don't really believe it." On a conscious level, this may be true, but in the television induced trance state these images have direct access to our subconscious and impact us deeply, particularly with repetition over time. There is a cost. We can say that we know we are not the mind and most thoughts are worthless, yet if our behavior doesn't support this, if we give our thoughts a lot of attention, is that really true?

The Truth about Emotional Eating

If your goal is to wake up out of the ego, why are you spending so much time living in this egoic world? In life, keeping good company is important. If you want to be happy and fulfilled, then set limits on how much time you spend feeding on mental junk food by sitting in front of the television.

Healing Emotional Eating

Ultimately, healing emotional eating is about learning how to tolerate feelings. We label these things "feelings" because we feel them in the body. You have thought, you believe it, and it takes root in your body. But rather than allowing yourself to be present with it, you have innocently formed the habit of distracting yourself from the feeling and seeking relief from it through instant pleasure. If, instead, you allow yourself to simply be present to the feeling rather than distracting yourself from it, you take an essential step in healing your emotional eating habit.

It's only through the actual experience of allowing a feeling to be present rather than running from it can you experience the truth about feelings rather than your conditioned reactions to them.

The next time an uncomfortable feeling arises try the following exercise:

Exercise – Healing Emotional Eating

To heal your emotional eating habit:

1. Practice seeing the whole truth about food.
2. Learn to tolerate feelings, rather than running from them. Whenever possible, find a quiet, private place to work with the feeling. Drop your story about whatever generated the feeling and simply allow the feeling to be present. Locate it in your body and focus on the sensation only. Allow the feeling to be there without any agenda for it to leave. Stay with it, until it dissipates.
3. Address what is off in your life. If you often feel sad or depressed, chances are your life is out of balance or you're spending most of your time engaged in activities that don't fit for you.
4. Question your stressful belief using inquiry. Feelings come from thoughts. If you're feeling bad, find out what you're thinking that caused you to feel this way. Then, use inquiry to see if that belief is really true. Here is an important rule of thumb. If a belief causes you to feel bad, it's never true.

What If We Have It All Wrong?

Most people are playing the game of life as if they read the rulebook. If you're going to play a game, the smart thing to do is to read the rules so you can strategize how to play to your best advantage. Similarly, in life if you understand the purpose behind it, you can plan your strategy.

What if the rules we learn from the culture that true happiness comes from amassing more stuff for "the me," like fame, riches, accomplishments, relationships were backwards. What if the notions of getting ahead, succeeding, making your mark were designed to lead us astray?

The values espoused by the culture are mirages. They are all trumped up and don't deliver. No wonder we get frustrated and try to get happy with food! In the next exercise, take an opportunity to travel to the end of your life and then allow the wisdom you bring back from this experience to inform your current life.

End of Life Meditation

Imagine that it's the end of your life and you have just breathed your last breath, and effortlessly and painlessly your body drops away. It feels like being released from a tightly fitting garment. At long last you're free! Imagine travelling down a long shimmering tunnel toward a warm welcoming white light. It's almost as if the light is connected to your own heart. It's beckoning, emanating unconditional love for you. You feel yourself effortlessly floating toward this light.

You have just crossed over into the dimension after death. Angels and your life helpers are there to greet you and welcome you. As you do your life review, you discover something truly remarkable. The so-called currency, the values ascribed to things in this astral world are completely different than the benchmarks in the life you just left. In other words the purpose of life on earth is completely different than what you thought it was.

You discover that what was valued by society was nothing more than culturally sanctioned conditioning. Accomplishment, achievement, possessions, the amount of money you have in the bank, a youthful, beautiful face and body, being admired for your appearance and accomplishments, numbers or friends and acquaintances, professional degrees and accolades, all of the things that were so revered in the life you just left, none of those things mattered. Our societal benchmarks for success were irrelevant.

Food, Freedom, and Truth

In other words, life has been a shell game, a world where nothing is what it seems and all of the things that seem valuable, are worthless and irrelevant and all of the things that get overlooked or seem inconsequential, are the only things that matter.

What if the ultimate lesson in this life were about love? What if we all came into this life with an outline – we had certain planned experiences and circumstances to help us learn about what was truly valuable? What if life were about expressing our gifts and talents, enjoying ourselves, valuing and deepening in the experience of our true nature—unbounded love and freedom? What if life were about putting love first, before being right or winning? What if life were about making love the most important thing? What if life were about waking up to our true identity as spiritual beings and expressing that through our human bodies?

THE TRUTH ABOUT HAPPINESS

If the mind is happy, not only the body but the whole world will be happy. So one must find out how to become happy oneself. Wanting to transform the world without discovering one's true self is like trying to cover the whole world with leather to avoid the pain of walking on stones and thorns. It's much simpler to wear shoes.

Ramana Maharshi

The more attention you give to your thoughts, the more you will experience discontentment and unhappiness. The more you turn away from your negative thoughts, the happier you will be. It's that simple.

Gina Lake

What World Do You Want to Live in?

In life you can choose to live in two very different worlds: the world of negative thoughts and feelings and the world of direct experience, peace, and contentment. Through your conscious attention, you choose your world.

The worldly currencies of wealth, reputation, and family connections cannot grant entrance to the world of peace and contentment. With no external gatekeepers, most people live unaware that their choice of world is completely under their control. And because these worlds are rarely referenced, most people are oblivious to the impact of their unconscious choice.

Experiencing life through the veil of negative thoughts and feelings means that stress and disconnection from life and others predominate. No one condemned you to this hell world. You create your own suffering when you put your attention on and believe in your negative thoughts. Christening a negative thought with belief generates negative feelings such as sadness, fear, despair, or anger. When this happens, you merge with the belief and feeling. For all practical purposes, you're the sadness, fear, or anger and the belief that spawned it. Consequently, you experience life at the negative thought's effect.

As human beings, we were programmed to identify with our negative thoughts. As a child growing up, you looked around and most people believed their negative thoughts and created negative feelings. Perhaps it never occurred to you that you had a choice or that your life could be different.

Turning your attention away from negative thoughts lands you in a heavenly world. Your life may occupy the same space,

The Truth about Happiness

with the same job, relationships, and physical address as your original hell world, yet your experience of life couldn't be more different. When you're identified with and give your attention to essence, the desire for food (or anything else for that matter) can't touch you. It has no power. It's like trying to flip on a light switch, when your power has been shut off. There is no juice and nothing happens.

From this place of essence, you may notice a budding desire arising in the form of the thought "I want." Yet if you don't give it your attention, if you turn away from it, it can't sprout into a full-blown desire with its anxiety producing, compelling need for fulfillment.

Therefore, the difference between happiness and unhappiness is completely a function of attention. Now that you know this is how life works, what world will you choose? Where will you put your attention? How you answer makes all the difference. As Robert Frost wrote: Two roads diverged in a wood, and I—I took the one less traveled by, and that has made all the difference.

What Are You Loving?

When it comes to your spiritual evolution, "Where is your attention right now?" is the most important question you can ever ask. Whatever you focus your attention on is what you're loving. If you're paying attention to a negative thought and believing it, you're loving that. When you pay attention to anything other than thoughts or feelings, you're aligned with essence, loving that, and therefore asking to experience more of that.

Life always honors that evolutionary impulse to know the truth. When we are loving essence with our attention, life delivers more experiences of truth and freedom. Eventually, something ticks over and we find that living from this place is completely natural. There is an irreversible seeing and once and for all, our true self is realized.

The greatest gift you can give someone is not an expensive present or money, but your undivided attention. Can you move outside of yourself, outside of your preoccupation with "me," what I like, what I want, or what I need, to focus on someone else? Can you be completely present with others and really see them?

It's easy to say, "Oh of course I can give my attention fully to someone else." Yet, if you actually try it, you may discover just how challenging it can be. After a short while, your mind will start to wander because placing your attention outside of yourself goes against your programming. Your default position, due to your conditioning, is to keep your attention fixed on yourself.

The Truth about Happiness

If you doubt this, notice how often you find yourself with people who are totally self-absorbed and can't seem to stop talking about themselves. If you're like most people in this situation, you can't wait to redirect the conversation back to yourself. They, on the other hand, will be reveling in this opportunity to have you join them in their interest in themselves.

To give another person your undivided attention requires a great deal of spiritual maturity. In the next day or two, notice how present you're with other people. When you give your complete attention to another person, by listening to them, without thinking of how you will respond or when you will be able to move the conversation back to your favorite subject, you, you're truly loving them.

Human programming keeps us locked into the "I thought," identifying as a person with a life and problems that need to be addressed. When we are distracted by situations in our lives, and decisions that we need to make, we aren't interested in asking the deeper questions like "who am I?" or "what am I doing here?" These deeper questions rock the boat of the false identity or ego and threaten to expose the illusion for what it's. It's therefore much better, from the ego's perspective, to keep us away from pondering such questions.

The downside of staying absorbed in "me" and "my life," is that it keeps you contracted and unhappy and reaching for food to give you some relief. This is counterintuitive. Wouldn't you think that focusing on yourself would have the opposite effect? Yet, ironically, if you look at the times in your life when you were the happiest, you were completely out of your head, and caught up in what you were doing. Thus, happiness and thinking about yourself are mutually exclusive states of consciousness. So, if you really want to be happy and heal your relationship with food, set the intention to keep your attention off of yourself. Don't touch any thoughts that start with the word "I." Focus instead on the experience you're having and you won't be able to avoid the joy and peace that envelops you.

Exercise – Ducking the "I" Thought

Set the intention to notice the thoughts you have that start with the word "I." Each time you notice such a thought, turn away from it. Similarly, when you notice thoughts that are about yourself, how something affects you or your life, turn away from it.

Being Present with Food

The first step in becoming more conscious in your relationship with food is bringing awareness to the situations and circumstances that you find yourself in when the idea of eating arises, assuming that you're not hungry.

When you feel the impulse to reach for food when you're not hungry and it's not time to eat, here is what I suggest:

Exercise – Inquiry When Urge to Eat Arises and It's Not Time to Eat

Delve a bit deeper. Ask yourself, "What am I thinking and feeling when the idea of eating arises?" Then, record these thoughts and beliefs in your journal. What do you notice about them? Are they part of a recurring stressful story that you've been telling yourself? Then, debunk the stories that you find using inquiry.

Next bring more awareness to your actual sensations of eating:

Exercise – Being Present with Sensation While Eating

Are you present with the sensations or are you so caught up in thinking and feeling, interacting with others, multi-tasking, driving, watching TV, or reading that you barely notice the experience of eating? What are the actual sensations of eating?

What does the food smell like? Taste like? Notice the temperature and texture of the food. How does it feel to chew it and swallow it?

Here are some suggestions to help you become more present when you're eating:

Exercise – Eating Awareness Tips

1. Begin by setting the intention and asking for help to be more present, more aware when you're eating.
2. Set aside time to eat alone without combining it with other activities. I call this "eating while you're eating."
3. Decide that eating is a "sitting down" activity and commit yourself to breaking the habit of eating while driving or standing up. So much unconscious, automatic eating happens when we're standing up, eating just a nibble here and a nibble there. When you want to eat something make sure to put the food on a plate and then sit down at a table and eat it.

The Ego's Relationship to Eating

Like an impatient toddler, the ego has a hard time delaying gratification. It ego would rather have a trivial, short-lived pleasure right now rather than wait for a more satisfying one later. Because eating is so pleasurable and because it satisfies a basic human need, our relationship with food give us an opportunity to get a great view of the inner workings of the ego.

Ironically, even though the ego is geared toward pleasure seeking and pain avoidance, when it obtains the object of its desire, rather than savoring the pleasure, it wants to get to the end of the experience as soon as possible.

When it comes to food, the ego wolfs it down at a dizzying speed. Table manners were invented in part to counteract the ego's tendency to eat like a half-starved animal. Ironically, even though the ego tries to keep us focused on pleasure seeking, the frenzied, unconscious eating that happens when we eat from the ego avoids the pleasure that eating was designed to provide.

One of the ego's favorite tactics is to keep us looking toward the future. Focused on results rather than experience, its objective is to get to the end of experiences as soon as possible. Then, when it reaches the end of the experience, it's sad that it's over. There is no pleasing the ego.

With all the hoopla it makes over striving to fulfill its desires, you would think that the ego would relish the pleasure when it wins the object of its desire. But when it comes right down to it, it has no interest in pleasure, anymore than it's interested in being present for any experience. Holding the object of its desire in its hands becomes like a game of hot potato. The ego's new goal is to get rid of it as fast as it can by rushing to the end of the experience.

The ego, doesn't feel the satisfaction that eating was designed to bring because it sidesteps the whole experience. And then feeling unsatisfied, it keeps us cramming more food into our mouths, trying to squeeze the pleasure out of the experience that it has sidestepped by rushing to finish whatever is on the plate.

Although the ego creates desires and cravings and luring us with promises of future pleasure, the ego is really a pleasure avoider. It avoids the pleasure of eating by:

- Voraciously gobbling it's food down
- Going unconscious, avoiding the sensation of eating and moving into the world of thoughts and feelings instead
- Denying the whole truth of overeating pleasure food: There is always a point when pleasure turns into pain.

Essence, on the other hand, is process oriented, more interested in enjoying the ride than in outcomes. Fascinated by each new experience, it takes its time, focusing all of its attention on whatever is appearing before it.

Essence, eats slowly and savors the food. It engages all of the senses, taking in the texture, temperature, taste, and smell of each bite. By bringing awareness to each moment, it actually prolongs and intensifies the pleasure of eating. If we are eating more slowly, we have time to pay attention and drop into the sensory experience of eating.

When we try to prolong the pleasure, however, we can overeat and the pleasure turns into pain. As a result, essence is present and awake to this turning point and stops eating prior to it to avoid causing the body discomfort. See if you can stay awake to this as well. In general, stop eating based on calories or portion size. However, if you begin to feel full prior to finishing your allotted portion, stop at this point instead.

If we enjoy the ride, if we are present and take the time to savor our food and experience the pleasure that eating was designed to give us, we feel satisfied at the end of the meal and don't need to try to prolong the experience by eating more.

It can take awhile to change the ego's habit of wolfing down its food. If you have rushed your eating and been aligned with the ego during the meal, there is no need to beat yourself up about it. At the end of the meal, you can simply notice the ego's discontent and consciously choose to be grateful instead. This choice drops you into essence and frees you from the ego's perpetual wanting.

Playing

Why is it that when we were kids, many of us dreaded being called in for dinner and now we relish any opportunity to put something good tasting into our mouths? How did food rise from the bottom to the top of our priority list, becoming our coveted favorite while we weren't looking?

Was life just more interesting when we were kids? Was playing so much better than the pleasures available to us as adults? In a word, yes. As kids we loved playing because it was how we connected with the present moment, with essence. When we're playing we're literally out of our heads with joy! We were reveling in this chance to experience life directly, as it was unfolding in the moment. That's why we love games.

Then we grow up and get serious lives and jobs and forget how to play. Finding ways to bring play back into our lives is one of the best things we can to do to free ourselves from eating and weight issues. Anything that moves us into essence weakens all of the egoic characters: the pleasure seeking child, the critic, and the dreamer. The characters encourage us to let them run our lives, assuring us that if we follow their instructions to a tee, true happiness awaits us. But the pleasures they lure us with are all trumped up and don't deliver. Not only don't they last, even when we gain the object of our desires, such as taste pleasure, riches, or beauty, they always bring suffering on their coat tails.

One of the best ways to escape from ego-based suffering is devoting ourselves to activities that align us with essence.

The Truth about Happiness

Whatever feels like play is likely to move you into the present moment and just like when you were a child, you too won't want to come in for dinner. Dancing, singing, listening to great music, painting, meditating, play acting, are just a few ways to move you out of your head and into your heart.

Support

Finding others committed to overcoming their eating and body image issues who are willing to support you in your journey can be a crucial arrow in your healing quiver. Not only can a support network speed up your healing, its very presence undermines the ego's insipid message that you're the only human being who struggles with food and weight.

In the past, the critic may have cruelly insinuated that you alone were spineless, weak-willed, and couldn't control this most basic of urges. But now, armed with your new support network, you can casually dismiss the critic's toothless judgments because the very existence of others who struggle with food negates them.

The people in your support network can relate to your struggles and commiserate with suffering that comes with so-called missteps and backslides that are often part and parcel of the journey. They can do this either because they've been there and done that, or because, just like you, they are in the process of becoming free themselves.

When I suggest creating a support network, I don't mean that you need a posse of eating police. Rather, find supportive compassionate people, like yourself, who have traversed the same eating terrain and want to become free. They need to understand your struggle from the inside out and know how to give gentle guidance and support. People who judge you and think that you're weak or believe that you should be able to just tough this through by getting a handle on yourself and getting on with it, need not apply.

The Truth about Happiness

You need lovers not scolders. Remember, the truth is always kind and words that come from essence are always kind. Scolding and admonishing are not kind.

It's likely that scolding, judging, and blaming have been your intimate acquaintances for quite some time now and you don't need more exposure to them or more practice. To heal you need to turn yourself around and move in the opposite direction. Renounce the ego's harsh tactics and instead practice kindness and compassion on the inside as well as the outside.

Let's get back to creating your support group. When it comes to supporters, quality trumps quantity. Recognize that not everyone who is committed to healing will be helpful to you. Choose someone who is wishes to change their relationship with their thought and not simply go on a diet. In other words, if your new supporter tells you that all you have to do is listen to your body when it comes to your eating choices and portion size run for the hills!

The Pleaser Disease

How can you know if you've been infected with the pleaser disease? Here are some questions to help you figure it out. Do you often find yourself doing things that you really don't want to do, saying "yes" when you really mean "no?" Do you give up something you want so that other people can have what they want? Is your mantra, "Whatever everyone else wants to do is fine with me"? If any of this sounds familiar, do you imagine that these "others" will repay your sacrifice by thinking well of you? Do you expect that they will like you more because you anticipated their needs and desires and did your best to fulfill them? If you answer, "yes" to any of these questions, do not "pass go," proceed immediately to the inquiry in the rest of this article to route out the pleaser disease.

The pleaser disease derives its momentum from fear. In the pleaser role, we create a story that includes scary, imagined consequences for daring to do what we really want to do or not doing what we think others want us to do.

Knowing that you're infected with the pleaser disease is the first step in healing it. If you're asked to do something, and you feel obligated to say "yes" when you really want to say "no," just because you think someone won't like you or will think less of you, realize that in that moment you're "people-pleasing," and tell yourself the truth about the consequences. Seeking the good opinions of other is a prescription for misery because:

1.   You feel bad

2. Feeling bad tends to send you running to the refrigerator

3. In spite of all of your pleasing antics, people don't necessarily like you or respect you any more for it.

If, you've been a people pleaser for most of your life, your seemingly selfless strategy comes with strings attached. Pleasers are sweet and nice on the outside but angry folks on the inside. In most cases, just beneath the surface, you resent the people you're trying to please. The reason for this is, in your pleasing endeavors, you subjugate your own needs and wants based on expectations that you attribute to them. This causes you to feel angry and resentful. Often this resentment surfaces as passive aggressive jabs broad-siding the poor, unsuspecting people out of nowhere!

Many of us who have eating issues have a hard time saying "no." As a result, we end up in situations that we don't want to be in. Then we stew about it, get upset at others and ourselves about it, and voila, we've set the stage for an eating explosion.

Look at how pleasing causes you to suffer and consider choosing differently from now on. Perhaps you don't need to go on that second family vacation with your in-laws. Maybe you don't need to host the church potluck. Is exposing yourself to an uncomfortable or unpleasant situation, an "Achilles heel" situation or person really necessary?

If food is your primary escape and you're a pleaser to boot, then I'll wager that people pleasing is one of the driving forces behind your emotional eating. One way to get your power back and stop creating the anger that's driving your eating is asking yourself, "What's the worst thing that could happen if I begin to assert myself and say "no" in situations where I might have said "yes" in the past? Will life as I know it end?"

Inquiring about the worst possible scenario and coming up with concrete possibilities, rather than amorphous potentialities, you see the truth rather than the ego's overblown fears about what would happen if you didn't people please. When you question the fears it's like turning on the light in a dark room and realizing that there are no zombies hiding under your bed. If you see that not only aren't the potential consequences catastrophic, but you can actually live with them, it gives you the latitude to experiment with "not pleasing" for a change.

Recognize that people's judgments about you're their problem, not yours. So let loose and begin to exercise your "no" muscle! If I were a betting woman, I would wager that there won't be much fallout from this new "non-pleasing" posture. Even if there is, ultimately, speaking your truth from a place of essence rather than ego is always in everyone's best interest.

The cure for Pleaser Disease is awareness, recognizing this pattern and coming to see:

1. It's okay to honor your own needs and preferences
2. You don't need to prove anything to yourself or others.

Healing the pleaser disease means becoming aware of your behavior and its impact on you and your relationships. Once you become more conscious, you have the freedom to choose, but from a place of seeing the whole truth about costs and benefits of this pattern. Rather than being run by unconscious fears and old habits, you can operate from what is fresh, alive, and true.

Essence is ever-present and moving you in this moment. When you're aware of it and choose to live from this place, life is joyous. You wake up out of suffering. Rather than being tethered to past ideas or patterns, you respond naturally to situations based on what feels true for you. This is the ultimate cure for the pleaser disease.

Asking for Support

Sometimes the people closest to us can unwittingly become our saboteurs. Without realizing it they become the accomplices of our critic, child, or dreamer. Their honey-tongued entreaties can be the speed bumps on our path toward a stable natural body weight and improved health.

They personify our critic, putting us down for wanting to improve our health because they naturally imagine themselves in our shoes, doing what we are doing, and for the most part, they don't want to go there. And because they're not willing, ready, or able to follow our lead, they resent us for making them look bad. They think, "Oh darn, if you're doing it, that means, I should do it too. And I don't want to go there! Ugh." Hence they want to get as far away from us as possible.

The other stand they can take is to embody our pleasure-seeking child. If we're hell bent on getting healthier and changing our relationship with food, they'll be damned if they'll sit back passively as we take this journey. They know they don't want to go, so they're determined to ply us with irresistible edibles until we fall off our wagon and land bloodied and discouraged on ours.

Finally, they can don the dreamer's guise, supporting our goal but for egoic reasons. "Oh yes, darling you have such a beautiful face, if only you could lose the weight, the world would be your oyster. There is nothing you couldn't do or get!" This could be a parent who liked to live vicariously through our successes. If we live the dream, they imagine that they are right there along with us. But the truth is, being admired or becoming someone else's arm candy is the booby prize.

The Truth about Happiness

Having the right size body, not only doesn't guarantee happiness, it's a surefire way of leading us down a path paved with suffering. People don't fall in love with bodies. They fall in love with authentic people whose tender hearts and souls open their own hearts.

That being said, if you live with people whom you feel have your health and best interest at heart, by all means, tell them what you're doing and ask for their support. People do love to help. If they care about you, they will welcome this opportunity to serve your growth and evolution. You do them a favor as well. There is nothing more gratifying than being of service to someone else.

The Short Cut to True Happiness

Don't tell the ego this, but there is a happiness that is different from the excited, giddy happiness that come from driving your new car home, winning at Bingo, or biting into a gooey brownie. It comes from being fully engaged in what you're doing and living in the present moment. We dip into this restful feeling of contentment several times a day, perhaps without even being aware of it.

The ego tells you that you have to do something to earn happiness and love. According to the critic and dreamer, these are prizes we attain only after steadfastly performing the arduous tasks it prescribes. Their strategy works something like this. First, the critic tells you about all the things that are wrong with you and makes you feel terrible. It tells you that you have to lose those 10, 20, or 200 pounds first. You have to heal your food issue or get your head together before anyone one else would want you. Then the dreamer steps in, offering salvation from the mess you're in. Sometimes we bypass the critic altogether and move straight to the dreamer setting lofty goals like getting a promotion or a doctorate first. Once you fulfill the task, others will notice how magnificent you're, and you will get all of the trappings of a happy life—the right partner, clothes, house, possessions, bank account and admiration and respect to win the brass ring called happiness.

The critic/dreamer approach to finding happiness looks convincing, particularly if you watch liquor commercials or read popular culture magazines. Our culture is the mouthpiece of the ego, espousing the same values. When we don't follow this course, we seem out of step with the rest of the world. We don't fit in and that can feel a bit uncomfortable. After all, we see everyone else doing it and they can't all be wrong, right?

The pleasure seeking child has another approach altogether. It tells you, "The critic and the dreamer want you to do so much work to get your slice of happiness. Forget those guys. Why not give yourself some pleasure right now. Why not just buy that new watch or dress? Why not dig into that pint of jamoca almond fudge ice cream? You can have happiness right now, rather than working so hard and waiting for. Come on. You deserve some pleasure right now!"

The ego is like the fake cop in the heist movie, who tells the real cops, "They went thatta way!" pointing them in the wrong direction. Or "Hurry up and get your happiness, it's this way!" "Just do as I say and happiness will be all yours for the rest of your life."

The only problem with this approach is that the ego, just like the crooked cop, is leading you in the wrong direction. It's leading you away from the moment and away from yourself, the true sources of happiness. This movement away will never yield the happiness that we all yearn for.

It's not surprising that we've fallen for the ego's tricks. We are programmed to pay attention to and follow our desires, taking action that will lead to their fulfillment. We get even more sucked into the ego's approach to life because when we follow the critic and dreamer's advice, for example, and get the svelte body or the promotion, we feel an excited kind of happiness. We delight in the belief, "Wow, I've finally arrived. I've finally made it and I will get the life I've always dreamed of."

But here is where our misunderstanding comes in. We feel great momentarily because we are no longer experiencing desire—suffering over not having what we want. We stop suffering over desire and we give the credit to the promotion or svelte body.

Then two things happen. First the ego gets bored and plants the seed for the next desire. It convinces you that it's time to move on to the next task. It says, "Okay we did that, now what?" It takes the massive effort or accomplishment for granted. So much for life long satisfaction and happiness! Second, you experience the fallacy of the dreamer's promise of a perfect life filled with everything you have always wanted and none of the things you don't want, now that you have reached your goal of a new slim body. Unlike your fantasies, your new body doesn't provide entrée into a dream life devoid of problems and challenges. Life is still life, beyond the ego's control, filled with surprises and unexpected difficulties.

When you have suffered enough to realize that the ego's values and strategies don't deliver happiness after all, but bring a feeling of emptiness and misery instead, perhaps you're ready to take the short cut to happiness.

The first step to avoid falling into the ego's trap is seeing the ego for the trickster it's. When the ego comes up with another brilliant plan, rather than falling under the familiar spell, you wake up and recognize that it's just the ego tempting you once again. It's not the wise part of you that knows better. This time you say "thanks but no thanks."

Instead, you choose differently, taking the short cut to happiness this time. Rather than follow the ego's plan that leads away from happiness, you feel into what is present in the moment, that vibrant aliveness that envelops you when you move out of thoughts and feelings and pay attention to everything else that is arising in the moment: the leaf floating

The Truth about Happiness

on the breeze, the warmth of the sun on your face, the sound of the bus as it goes by, the feeling of your breath moving in and out of your body, the smell of coffee brewing next door.

The direct experience of whatever is present right now is the short cut to happiness. When you notice yourself getting caught up in thought and worry ask yourself, "Where is the quiet?" This simple question will bring you into the present moment and your natural state of happiness. The ego will try to convince you that this is preposterous, way too simple. Instead it will try to hook you with its seductive sounding plans and in this way, keep you circling around happiness and never quite landing there.

Like Moses prohibited from entering the promise land, the ego can't ever enter the present moment and as a result can't experience true happiness. So rather than filtering experience through the mind, which can be like observing your meal through a plate glass window or reading a description of it rather than eating it, you ignore your minds suggestions and instead, sink into the happiness that is always available, free, and requires nothing of you.

Four Ways To Weaken Conditioning

Unknowingly, most of us live under the unconscious influence of debilitating beliefs that we formed in childhood. When they get triggered, these same beliefs cause us to sprint toward the refrigerator. We innocently created these beliefs to protect ourselves from situations similar to the ones that caused us to create the conditioning in the first place. But now, as adults we realize that this conditioning is holding us back and keeping us from living fully and freely.

When you were young, if a parent or classmate made fun of you, you might have decided to hang back and not to put yourself out in the world. In this way, you avoided situations that could bring up uncomfortable shameful feelings such as these. Whether you realize it or not, that conditioning has continued to dictate how you live, the risks you take or don't take, who you approach for romance or friendship, the career choices you make or don't make and on and on.

As an adult, living constrained by your fear-based conditioning creates a certain repression of life. There is a way in which you're not following your heart because fear is blocking you from doing what is true for you in the moment. It's hard to be happy if you're not living aligned with your life purpose. And how can you align with your life purpose when unconscious fears are putting up roadblocks to doing and saying what is true for you? So where does this leave you? What do you do? Simple: you put one foot in front of the other and begin to uncover and heal your conditioning.*

Here are four ways you can heal conditioning:

Exercise – Four Ways to Heal Your Conditioning

If our core beliefs are unconscious, ask for help to be able to see them. Ask that they bubble up to consciousness. Then pay attention. You may be in a restaurant and overhear someone saying something at the table next to you or be struck by a line in a song that triggers a memory or belief.

* Once you uncover a dormant belief, take it to inquiry.
1. Is it true?
2. Can you absolutely know that it's true?
3. How do you react, what happens, when you believe that thought?
4. Who would you be without the thought?

Then, turn around the concept you're questioning to its opposite, and be sure to find at least three genuine, specific examples of each turnaround.

* When a feeling arises just let it be there. Drop any story you have about it and just focus on the sensation that is manifesting in your body. Don't have an agenda for it to leave. Just let the feeling do it's dance. Get very still and absorb yourself in the sensation. Then, notice the insights that arise. If the insights contain any stressful beliefs, take them to inquiry.

* Notice a stressful thought and catch it before an emotion is created. You have to be quick for this one. Thoughts generate emotions, almost instantaneously. But it's possible to catch a thought before it creates a negative emotion and either: Ignore it or debunk it through inquiry

* Spending lots of time in essence weakens conditioning. This is the indirect path to healing conditioning and a great support to the process. The more time you spend in essence aligned

with your heart instead of the thinking mind, the less most thoughts hold any fascination for you. Conditioning is made up of thoughts. If you're ignoring stressful thoughts, then your conditioning crumbles and stops covering over your happiness.

The Truth about Happiness

The great news is using any or all of these four strategies can free you. You don't need to live out the rest of your days in the prison of your conditioning. Even though we were all programmed to create conditioning, you came equipped with your very own "break out of jail card" in the form of consciousness. As soon as you ask for help, set the intention to live from a freer place, and put one of these four strategies into practice, you start the process of moving out of suffering and into a happier way of living.

* A great book about healing conditioning is *Getting Free: How To Move Beyond Conditioning And Be Happy* by Gina Lake. www.radicalhappiness.com

**For more information, about Byron Katie and The Work, go to www.thework.com

A Gratitude Attitude

I'm not a betting woman, but if I were to take odds, I'd guess that your ego doesn't have many nice things to say about your life. However lousy its complaining makes you feel, this negativity serves its plan. Here is your ego's pitch, "if you don't like your life, leave it to me, your good friend the ego, to fix. Enter my mental world, and hang out in the exotic fantasies about the future, that I will help you create, where life will conform to your preferences."

Rather than seeing the whole picture of what is arising right now, the ego wants to accentuate the negative sliver of truth about what is appearing in the present moment. It's very clever. How better to keep you out of direct experience, out of the now, than to tell you it stinks and build a case for that? To stay in charge of your life and keep you identified as a limited, fragile body-mind, it's better to engage you in the let's pretend game, weaving grandiose images of an imagined future.

The only problem with this strategy is: you miss life. Life is always happening now. There's only this moment and if you miss it, there's no going back. Fortunately, no matter how bleak the ego's characterization, there are always things to appreciate about what's arising right now. If you're not seeing the positive, you're not looking hard enough.

We're programmed to listen to ego's complaints about life. We're born kvetchers, but we don't have to live that way. Take a moment right now and list three things you appreciate about your life. Then, list three qualities that you appreciate about this moment. They can be small things. After all that's really where the juice or rasa is. Here are some examples:

I love:

The Truth about Happiness

1. Seeing the sun peering from behind the cloud.
2. Feeling the breeze on my skin.
3. The sensation of aliveness in this body.
4. Having the use of my arms and legs.
5. Feeling my breath moving in and out of my body.
6. Seeing these words that I'm reading.

If you don't believe that egos are programmed to be negative, look around you and notice whatever is in your immediate environment. Pretty soon you will find yourself judging, lamenting, or complaining. "The lamp could be a little brighter," "How did that table get dusty already?" "The heat isn't working properly in this room. Why couldn't they have designed the heating system to be more efficient."

Now notice your thoughts when you're talking to someone else or leafing through the mail: "Gosh, listen to how she just goes on and on." Can't she just say it in a sentence rather than going on for five minutes about it." "Why are there always so many bills and so few checks?" Notice how contracted these thoughts make you feel.

This habitual way of approaching life is not you, not the real you, anyway. It's just egoic conditioning in action. The ego views the world through the perspective of lack. If you really want to turbo charge your evolution, change the prescription of your glasses. See the world as supporting you, giving you exactly what you need in every moment. What if every experience had a gift for you and it was your job to find it?

Life may not always feel good, but where is written that it has to? Clearly, even the suffering serves a purpose—teaching us to make choices that move us toward, rather than away from love.

Food, Freedom, and Truth

It's said that all of the celestial beings in heaven envy human beings because it's only in a human body that one can experience the truth. Remember this. Be grateful for the gift of this human body and your good fortune, rather than complaining about what you don't have. If you don't have something or if you lost something, you didn't need it.

As an antidote to the negative, glass half empty way that the ego looks at life, I recommend adopting a gratitude practice. Like meditation, it's a powerful spiritual practice that will wake you up out of the ego's programing and serve your spiritual growth. Take out your journal and make a list of twenty things you're grateful for. Even if your lover has just left you, one of your parents died last week, and you just lost your job, there are still many things in your life and in everyday experiences to be grateful for. We take so many of life's gifts for granted: the sunrises and sunsets, the variability of the weather, trees beginning to bud in the springtime, breathing, food, clothing, a roof over our heads.

The more you can practice gratitude, the happier you will be and the less likely you will be trying to get happy by cramming chocolate chip cookies into your face. In this way, you cultivate a positive mind and consciously reverse your old habit of a negative posture toward life. You stop eating to avoid the negativity in your own mind.

> ### Exercise – Gratitude
>
> Tomorrow, and each day forward for the rest of your life, when you first wake up, think of at least three things you appreciate about yourself and your life. Then, start your day.

Appreciation is a quality of essence. By starting your day in essence rather than in ego, you're awake to life's beauty and are less likely to seek after ego pleasures that leave you feeling flattened and unsatisfied. See what happens to your experience of life from beginning your day with this "gratitude attitude." Regardless of your life circumstances, your life can't help but become   easier   and   happier.

Guided Meditation

On so many levels, meditation is one of the best gifts you can give yourself. There is nothing like it to help you become happier and heal your emotional eating habit. Even if you can only set aside a few minutes each day to connect with essence through meditation, either guided or silent, you will transform your life.

In case you haven't noticed, your experience of life is your life! You either experience life directly or you experience it mentally based on how you think about it. Two people living parallel lives can have radically disparate inner experiences. One is blissful, identified with essence, while the other is miserable, identified with ego. It's the shifting of inner alignment from ego to essence, primarily through meditation, that makes all the difference.

In guided meditation, focusing on the guide's voice shifts you into receptivity, into listening, which requires humility. Because your ego thinks it knows everything, it hates to listen.. It could care less about what the other person is saying and can't wait to move the conversation back to its favorite topics: "Me," "What I want," "What I think," "What I like," and Why you should agree with me," etc.

Guided meditations are helpful for beginning a meditation practice because the sound of the guide's voice moves the meditator out of thinking into the present moment. Silent meditation, on the other hand, can be frustrating at first, because it often turns into a battle with the mind, which we can never win of course! Guided meditation sidesteps that vexing problem. And at the same time, it moves us into essence because we can't listen and think at the same time.

It almost doesn't matter what is being said or whether it's even in a language that we understand! This explains why prayers and chants in foreign languages can transport people as easily into essence as prayers and chants in their native language. Understanding happens through the mind and we actually don't need to understand something to align with our true nature. The experience of what we are is always available to us and lies just below that surface of thought.

Meditation helps to keep the wise part of us in charge. Here's how it works. When we meditate, we become accustomed to the delicious way we feel, and we allow that feeling, to flow into the rest of our lives. We become more comfortable with essence and when the ego comes back on the scene, it doesn't feel good to us at all! We become less willing to hang out in the egoic state and shift very quickly back to essence.

Whether we are identified with ego (the chatterbox in our heads) or essence (the peaceful undercurrent that flows through life) makes all the difference in our happiness and in our experience of life. When we're in essence, we feel good. It stands to reason that if we're happy, we won't feel a need to reach for food to comfort or entertain ourselves.

Unraveling the tangled yarn of our addictive relationship with food requires a mature and compassionate approach. The more we meditate, the more we're aligned with the wise, rational part of ourselves, the more we connect with the unending supply of love that is flowing through us all the time. When we are in this flow, we don't need any other relationship to be happy—not with lovers, friends, children, possessions, or food. We are being fed from the inside. From that place of self-sufficiency, peace, and joy, we come to each relationship clean, without demands or conditions, knowing that who we are doesn't need anything or anyone. Who we are and what we have is enough.

In summary, nothing weakens the ego and aligns us with essence like meditation. If you can commit to finding time in your schedule to give yourself that gift, I promise you that you will become happier, and more centered, resilient and consequently, more able to deal with life challenges in a balanced way, rather than reaching for food to numb out or distract yourself. (See Mind-BodyReset.com for guided meditation MP3 downloads.)

Accepting Resistance

The starting point for any transformation, whether it's inner or outer, is acceptance. To clear up a few misconceptions that have sullied its good name, let's start with what acceptance is not. It's not an affirmation. It's not pretending that you're okay with something when you're not by painting on a Pollyanna smile and saying, "Yes of course this is fine, when every bone in your body is screaming, "Hell no—no way!"

Often people confuse acceptance with liking something. Luckily you don't have to like your body to accept it. *You can actually move into acceptance by acknowledging that you don't like it.* Here is how it works: you accept the present moment— your body looks how it looks right now and you don't like its size or shape. Although you may well prefer a thinner body, the starting place for exchanging your current body for a thinner one is accepting the truth: your body is heavy *right now and you don't like it.* Six months from now, it may look different, but for right now, this is it.

Acceptance is acknowledging the truth of whatever is arising in the moment, whether it's an obese body or fear or the end of a relationship. This movement into acceptance is a strict gatekeeper, allowing through only the truth of what is so right now, while refusing entry to any fantasies about what we wish were so. It's telling ourselves the truth: "what is appearing in this moment is not my preference yet I accept it's reality."

Imagine being a reporter charged with dispassionately ascertaining the truth about a situation. All you care about is the facts, the "who, what, where, and when" of the present moment. True to your charge, you won't put up with any judgements, characterizations or airy, fairy ideas about what woulda, coulda, or shoulda been.

Like it or not, there is no way to change the present moment. It arises and passes away so quickly that before you can say, "this needs to be different now," that "now moment" has moved into the past. It's over.

Unless you're psychic, you can't know how your body will look in six months, a year, or ten years. However, if you want a healthier body, it's important to accept that you have the one you have now. You don't have to like it, just accept that this is the way your body looks now. To not accept its current state or appearance is denial.

This kind of no nonsense acceptance, even if it feels like resignation, is still acceptance. It's the acceptance of being in resistance to the way your body is appearing. When you can let it be okay that you don't like the way your body looks, something inside relaxes and you feel at peace. As confusing as it may sound, accepting resistance is still acceptance.

Once you accept the truth of this moment, you immediately drop into your true nature or essence. From essence, you're aligned with your own innate wisdom and connected with where life is moving you.

The flip side of acceptance is resistance. Have you heard the expression, "what you resist persists?" If you're busy railing at God and wishing that something else was happening, *other than what is happening*, essence can't get your attention. There is no room for the wise, creative part of you to inspire and move you into fruitful action.

When you're resisting the present moment and holding the resistance in place by denying the truth about it, you're caught in a cycle of judgment and self-hatred in your mind. You're stuck in ego and from this place it's next to impossible to take positive action.

Even though it seems counterintuitive, the first step in transformation is accepting the situation that you want to change. You accept your resistance to the undeniable existence of the very thing you don't want to have in your life. This acceptance of resistance moves you into essence. From essence you feel your way, sensing what is flowing inside of you and guiding your journey. From this wise, true place, rather from the ego's story of judgment and self-hatred, you discover what if anything you're motivated to do about a particular situation. Whether or not you feel moved to take action, the humility of telling yourself the truth about your resistance moves you into your heart and aligns you with essence. As soon as you move into essence your suffering ceases and clarity about the situation you have been resisting will soon follow.

Choice

Believing that we don't have choices in life makes it next to impossible to be happy. When we tell ourselves the story that we're locked into our lives with no way out, it's not surprising that we feel hopeless and depressed. We rationalize away our happiness by saying things like, "I have to keep working at this job until I put my kids through college" or "I have to hold out five more years until retirement" or " I really want to do X but I could never do that. What would people think of me?"

When we have this posture toward life, it's as if we've given ourselves a prison sentence, and now we're counting down the days until we can do what we really want to do. Living this way is more of a "dying" than a living. No wonder we turn to food to bring some pleasure to our dreary existence!

Yet how we experience life, how it feels to us, is based entirely on how we think about it. If we believe that we're blessed by our circumstances, the sun is shining, even in a heavy downpour, and we feel light and happy. If we believe we have no options, we feel doomed and powerless and day to day living feels like a chore.

If believing that we are trapped in our lives with no apparent way out, the negative feelings caused by our circumstances and this belief don't just vaporize; they have to go somewhere. We either repress them, take them out on other people (either through passive or overt aggression), feel miserable, create health problems, eat, or any combination of the above.

The ego is always looking to feel happy and comfortable and who could blame it? When it'sn't able to achieve this, it reaches for its addictive substance of choice. If we've seen food as our primary source of comfort, solace, and pleasure, we naturally reach for it, hoping to stuff down the sadness we created when we bought into the belief of being trapped in an unsatisfying life.

How do we escape this painful cycle? The first step is awareness. If you're not happy, ask yourself, "What story am I in? What am I telling myself to make me feel this way?" If you discover that you're telling yourself the story of "no choice," you can know, right off the bat that this is a lie. The circumstance called "no choice" is never the case because life always has options.

Most importantly, there are "thinking" options. Weaving a negative story makes you suffer, not just some of the time—but all of the time. When you really see this, victim-hood is erased from your vocabulary. You take responsibility for your state and become the ruler of your inner world.

Begin by challenging any limiting stories you've been telling yourself. If you've convinced yourself that you *have* to do continue doing what you hate, is that really true? You can't quit the job you hate. Is that true? You have other options. You can move somewhere with a lower cost of living, or get a different job more suited to you, or work for yourself doing something you love.

You choose to stay in the unhappy marriage. You choose to work for the abusive boss. You choose to live in the big, expensive house. You choose to work two jobs to pay for college, but you don't have to. Make your own happiness a priority. Do you believe that your child wouldn't be able to go to college without your efforts? Do you believe that you

Food, Freedom, and Truth

wouldn't be able to survive if you changed careers or quit the job that doesn't suit you?

You live a certain way because you have been choosing it. Unless you acknowledge this truth, you will feel powerless and unhappy. If you feel boxed in, ask yourself, "What are my options in this situation?" Open your mind. Don't let the critic come in with its vituperative commentary. Just live in this question: "If money weren't an issue and I could really do whatever I wanted to do, live the way I wanted to live, what would that look like?" For the moment, forget the consequences or what other people might think. When you open yourself to new possibilities in this way, you're available and open when they come knocking.

You may not choose to take steps that would lead you to a particular option today or tomorrow or ever. Yet there is great freedom and relief in knowing that you have the power to make that choice, if you want to. "I could do something different and I'm choosing to do what I'm doing, instead. At some point, I might choose differently, but for right now, I'm choosing this."

Fulfill Your Spiritual Destiny

As human beings we're programmed to feel that we aren't enough and we don't have enough. This programming keeps us perpetually striving to be more, and have more of what we think we need to be happy. The ego directs us to external solutions to our discontent like acquiring more skills, education, fame, a better appearance, a romantic relationship, more money, or even spiritual advancement. All of these serve to augment our sense of self, or so we think.

For those of us who have food issues our gnawing emptiness sends us to the refrigerator for to fill the hole in our souls. Our underlying assumption is: there is something outside of myself that can actually deliver this relief. The problem with external solutions to the ego's story of lack is that they ultimately turn out to be mirages. They satisfy or distract us for a few moments and then, either the old hole returns, or a new one opens up.

When I finally reached my goal weight, I spent all of a minute and a half reveling in my success before my ego began ruminating about the other problems in my life. The ego is in the problem creation and solution business. When you solve an egoic problem, you attain the object of your desire. Due to the cessation of this desire, you stop suffering.

From the ego's perspective, the end of suffering, even if it's momentary, sends it into a panic. Without suffering, without a problem to solve or the discomfort of a desire, you wake up out of identification with it and shift into essence. From essence there is no ego with problems that needs solving. Problems are its raison d'etre. Without them, it might as well retire and give up its illusion of controlling your life.

Not only can't the ego coexist with essence, moving there is synonymous with annihilation. When you're identified as essence, as the spiritual being that you have always been, the ego is dead to you. Like everything else, the ego doesn't want to die. It hangs onto its superior position in your life with bloody fingernails until you say, "I've had enough. I'm ready to stop suffering over food. I'm ready to wake up and fulfill my spiritual destiny."

If you're reading these words, it's very possible that reaching for food to fill up the hole in your soul is your path to the truth. That is the gift in your food misalignment. The beauty of this egoic drive for fulfillment is: like all egoic desires, it's a reflection of a deeper spiritual desire, essence's intention for you to return home. The emptiness you feel is rooted in a deeper need, a true need for connection with source—the only thing in life that truly feels satisfying.

Thankfully, food issues are excruciatingly painful. As odd as it may seem, this is another sign of life's mercy, of a friendly universe. The sheer agony of it means that you will look for a way out quickly and probably leave no stone unturned in your efforts to heal.

When you reach this point and you're tired of suffering, it may also mean that you're ready to move into deeper alignment with yourself. It's a sign that it's time to look within for the joy that your outer searching has obscured. Up until now, fixating on the glazed donut distracted you and caused you to assume that what you want and need exists somewhere outside of yourself.

The Truth about Happiness

Yet, once you reach the place in your evolution of seeing the futility of outward seeking, you move within through meditation, inquiry, reading spiritual books, going to spiritual gatherings, retreats or immersing yourself in creative pursuits. As you strengthen this inner connection with yourself, the world loses its ability to fool you with its story that you're a needy hole that needs filling. Thankfully, being centered in your own truth undermines both the world's power to scare you and to fulfill you. This is what the sages mean when they talk about moving beyond the world—being in it but not of it.

So rather than cursing your food issue and feeling like its victim, can you be grateful for it? If it leads you to liberation in this lifetime, would it all have been worth it? Reaching this crossroad and recognizing where everything in your life has been leading, use your food related suffering to propel you toward something greater. Use it to realize and fulfill the purpose of your life and come to know the truth about yourself. Use it to liberate yourself from all suffering and become the blessing to the world that you were meant to be.

Further Reading

A great book about healing conditioning is *Getting Free: How to Move Beyond Conditioning and Be Happy* by Gina Lake. www.radicalhappiness.com

For more information about Byron Katie and *The Work*, go to www.thework.com.

www.ingramcontent.com/pod-product-compliance
Lightning Source LLC
Chambersburg PA
CBHW072359290526
45794CB00001B/113